Paleo Diet Cookbook

The Ultimate Guide Of Paleo Diet To Cracked Weight Loss,

Be More Healthier And Improve Your Lifestyle

(Lose Up To One Pound Per Day)

By James Press

Introduction

Hi friend, this is James Press! Firstly, I would like to congratulate and thank you for choosing this book: *"**Paleo Diet Cookbook-The Ultimate Guide Of Paleo Diet To Cracked Weight Loss, Be More Healthier And Improve Your Lifestyle(Lose Up To One Pound Per Day)**"*.

Many people face the problem of being overweight! You may have tried various ways to cut fat, but the effect is BAD. You might lose weight during a diet, but only to have it return quickly. This yoyo effect of dieting is detrimental to the body. But this time, you will achieve an amazing effect by a Paleo diet. This book will solve the dieting dilemma for you.

Paleo diet is a form of diet which dates back to the times of our ancestors, and that is why it has been referred to as "**Caveman Diet**," **Stone Age Diet, or Primal Diet**! Paleo Diet is now more and more popular around the world, as it has too many benefits for our body health and weight loss. Usually we eat foods that are natural and without processed foods, which are same with the ones that antient people ate. We know the antients are strong and health, seldom have illness, that's why we explore this paleo diet world. University suggests that it is advisable for people who follow a Paleo diet to take 35% of their total calorie intake from fats, the rest from 35% from carbohydrates, and the final 30% from the proteins

When you follow Paleo diet, it is not just about **losing weight**. It will also make you **feel better, look better, have more energy, reduce pain, boost sex drive, prevent disease, and increase longevity**... and best of all, you will still be able to eat some of the foods you crave and achieve a slimmer body.

Get started now! This super Paleo diet book will **lead you to know everything about Paleo**. Why it is really effective? How to start? Most important mistakes you need to avoid! All you will know from here! Even in the next few weeks the results you will see in the mirror are going to be indisputable.

For the **110+ Paleo Diet recipes**, which are simple yet delicious and easy to make, we have provided the image, full nutrition values, and step-by-step directions how to make it.

The core purpose of this book is to not only allow you to fully understand the potential of a Paleo Diet, but to give you an awesome, delicious meal plan to kick start your Paleo journey! We have provided a **4-week Paleo diet meal plan**, which includes healthy and appetizing recipes. Each meal or recipe will also include nutritional values. Wish you will have a pleasant journey of Paleo Diet! So, don't wait up any longer and go ahead.

Table of Contents

Chapter 1: Essentials Of Paleo Diet

What Is Paleo Diet?

While there are hundreds of different kinds of diet regimes floating around, claiming to drastically alter the human physique and help an individual to trim down their body fat, very few of them are actually effective.

When counting the effective ones, Ketogenic Diet often comes to mind first. But, an extremely potent alternative, "The Paleo" diet is slowly climbing up the ladders of prosperity, where now it has turned into a total sensation amongst health buffs!

The main motto of this spectacular form of diet tries to answer a very simple question: "What was the diet of a caveman?"

We are basically trying to follow a modern evolutionary version of the diet which was followed by our ancestors.

The esteemed author of "The Paleo Diet", Loren Cordian professed that a Paleo Diet helps to lessen the amount of glycemic load and boasts a healthy ratio of saturated in comparison to unsaturated fatty acids, which further enhances the intake of nutrient and vitamins.

Is It Possible To Lose 30 Pounds In 4 Weeks?

One thing you should keep in mind is that a "Paleo Diet" is not a diet that directly helps to lose weight. Instead, it helps to encourage a healthy lifestyle which leads to a longer, healthier life.

But here's the catch, one of the primary effects of a Paleo diet, aside from increasing your longevity, is that it greatly encourages to lower the level of your fat. It encourages you to make the right choices in choosing your food and prevents you from consuming unhealthy condiments.

Assuming that you are absolutely new to the world of Paleo Diet, the following summarizes basic factors of Paleo Diet and weight loss:

- Always make sure to consume high-quality protein food with healthy fats in each meal. Make sure not to skip on these two thinking you might "save your calories" for future efforts
- Make sure to go for as many vegetables and fruits as you can. Consume at least one serving of fresh green plant in your meal.
- Just because your main goal is to lose your weight, make sure you don't starve yourself! For the Paleo diet to work properly, you are need to eat properly.
- Make sure to keep your Paleo diet mostly limited to meat or vegetables and try to avoid cookies or pancake type treats.

If you have started to follow these basic rules, then some of the immediate effects that you will observe will include:

- A rapid loss of 5-10 pounds the first couple weeks.
- After which, the rate of weight loss will taper slightly, to approximately 3-7 pounds per week.

Have a look at the graph below.

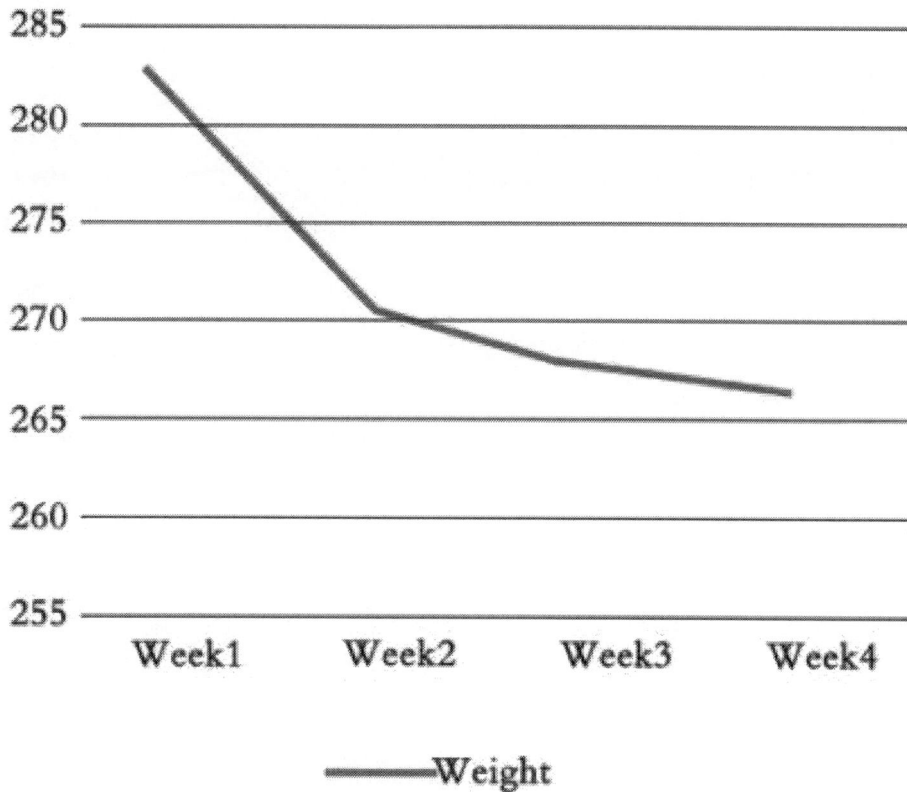

Illustration 1: Weight Graph

As people have different body health, shape, and body type it may not possible for a person to completely lose 30 pounds if you rely solely on a Paleo diet during 4 weeks, but it still gives you a steady flow of weight loss.

The Physiological Changes That Occur On A Paleo Diet

Following a Paleo Diet will bring about some changes to your body both on a cellular level and also on the large scale. To summarize:

- Paleo diet greatly aids in weight loss, albeit indirectly. The abundance of protein and fat in your body creates satiety which gives you a feeling of being full. The body meets up with the nutritional requirements of your body as a result you won't have to eat as much and as such, the body will start losing weight.

- The intake of amino acids and healthy fats from carbohydrates and proteins encourages carbohydrate metabolism which increases digestion.
- In terms of a physiological change, following a Paleo diet will increase your body to gain muscle, which is essential for individuals who may be underweight.
- The increased level of libido thanks to a more balanced weight will also affect the level of hormones in your body and balance them out to allow you to control your emotions and sexual drive.
- Having a Paleo diet will encourage your body to get more essential elements such as Omega 3 Fatty acids, B5, Selenium and even zinc 5, which helps to make your skin softer and clearer, and reduce chance of acne.
- If you are suffering from a tooth decay, then Paleo diet will help to get you away from a sugary diet that might cause damage to your enamel.
- Consuming more leafy vegetables, will help increase the level of Leptin that will encourage the level of fertility in your body.
- As a female on Paleo diet, you won't be consuming as much dairy products and caffeine, and could experience less cramping during your cycle.

The Myriad Of Benefits Coming From A Paleo Diet

Aside from helping to lower your body fat, Paleo diet helps by increasing the well-being of multiple aspects in your body. Some of these benefits are:

- Encourages health of your cells by properly balancing out the level of saturated and unsaturated fat.
- Paleo diet is packed with Omega-3 Fatty acids. DHA coming from Paleo Diet benefits your eyes, heart, brain function and development.

- Paleo diet helps your body gain essential vitamins and minerals, increases overall immunity, and health longevity.
- Paleo diet will reduce inflammation and decrease the chances of cardiovascular disease.
- Paleo diet will help you to become and remain energetic throughout the day.

Essential Tips For Starting Your Paleo Journey!

Now that you are properly aware of the benefits of Paleo and what Paleo is, I am sure you are excited to jump on the band wagon! But before you do, these tips are going to kick start your Paleo journey. Here are some tips:

- Properly separate food groups before eating. For example, a specific category for sugar followed by dairy, beans, wheat, and then legumes.
- Try to follow a 4-week challenge, such as the one in this book
- Before starting your journey, remove all the tempting (junk) foods from your kitchen
- Directly jumping on full Paleo diet might be tough. Start out slowly. Alternate an unhealthy snack with a healthy Paleo snack and slowly replace unhealthy items in your diet with healthy Paleo items.
- Make sure to do a thorough research before starting your Paleo diet
- If possible, detoxify your body before starting Paleo Diet. It will help you further
- Make sure to build up a nice, strong mentality. Prepare yourself to follow through the Paleo diet. Don't leave it halfway through, the journey to your goal might take some time, but you will achieve it.

List Of Foods To Eat/ Avoid During Your Paleo Diet

Paleo Diet is all about making sure you consume the right food. If you go astray, then things won't work out for you as good as they should. So, it is essential to keep a list of the do's and don'ts. Have a look below for a rough idea.

Foods To Eat

- Meats, including lamb, beef, turkey, chicken, pork
- Seafood, such as trout, haddock, shellfish
- Omega-3 enriched eggs
- Vegetables, including peppers, kale, broccoli, carrots, onions, etc.
- Fruits, including bananas, apples, pears, strawberries, avocados, blueberries
- Tubers, including sweet potatoes, turnips, yams
- Nuts and seeds, such as macadamia, almonds, walnuts, hazelnuts, sunflower seeds
- Fats and Oil, as coconut oil, avocado oil, olive oil
- Salt, such as himalayan salt, sea salt, turmeric, garlic, rosemary

Foods Not To Eat

- Items that are high in fructose or sugar such as drinks, candy, fruit juices
- Grain type items such as wheat, rye, barley
- Lentils
- Vegetable oil, corn oil, sunflower oil, soybean oil
- Hydrogenated products
- Artificial Sweeteners
- Heavily processed foods

Setting up proper goals for your Paleo journey

It is recommended to set a proper goal when you consider embarking on something, especially a diet. But at the same time, if you set your goals too high, then all of your hard work could be in vain.

In terms of Paleo, there are a few things which you should really keep in mind when setting up your goal. Basically, you are going to need to set realistic goals.

Off the top of my head, some things you should keep in mind include:

- Your ideal target for each week should be around 2 to 4 pounds.
- Patience is a virtue, and you should not aim to get slim and trim within a few days! It might take a few tries.
- While exercising is essential, you should not keep that a goal. If it is possible then you should go for it.
- Make sure to never skip breakfast. While trimming yourself down should be your goal, starving yourself is not recommended! Make sure to have breakfast, lunch, and dinner properly.

Let's have a look at something more specific.

Setting up your weight goal

Before setting the desired target weight, you should have a look at your Body Mass Index (BMI).

In simple terms, the BMI is a method of measurement which is done by comparing both the height and weight of a person in order to come out with a rough idea of the person's physique. The formula below is used to calculate the BMI of a person.

$$BMI = \frac{weight\ (\text{kg})}{height^2(\text{m}^2)}$$

$$BMI = 703 \times \frac{weight\ (\text{lb})}{height^2\ (\text{in}^2)}$$

Illustration 2: Body Mass Index

Once the Index has been obtained, a similar chart to the one below will enable you to assess the results.

BMI CHART

Weight lbs	100	105	110	115	120	125	130	135	140	145	150	155	160	165	170	175	180	185	190	195	200	205	210	215
kgs	45.5	47.7	52.3	50.0	54.5	56.8	59.1	61.4	63.6	65.9	68.2	70.5	72.7	75.0	77.3	79.5	81.8	84.1	86.4	88.6	90.9	93.2	95.5	97.7

Hight in/cm — 12-18 Underweight   18-24 Healthy   25-29 Overweight   30-39 Obese   40-42 Extremely Obese

Height																								
5'0"-152.4	19	20	21	22	23	24	25	26	27	28	29	30	31	32	33	34	35	36	37	38	39	40	41	42
5'1"-154.9	18	19	20	21	22	23	24	25	26	27	28	29	30	31	32	33	34	35	36	36	37	38	39	40
5'2"-157.4	18	19	20	21	22	22	23	24	25	26	27	28	29	30	31	32	33	33	34	35	36	37	38	39
5'3"-160.0	17	18	19	20	21	22	23	24	24	25	26	27	28	29	30	31	32	32	33	34	35	36	37	38
5'4"-162.5	17	18	18	19	20	21	22	23	24	24	25	26	27	28	29	30	31	31	32	33	34	35	36	37
5'5"-165.1	16	17	18	19	20	20	21	22	23	24	25	25	26	27	28	29	30	30	31	32	33	34	35	35
5'6"-167.6	16	17	17	18	19	20	21	21	22	23	24	25	25	26	27	28	29	29	30	31	32	33	34	34
5'7"-170.1	15	16	17	18	18	19	20	21	22	22	23	24	25	25	26	27	28	29	29	30	31	32	32	33
5'8"-172.7	15	15	16	17	18	19	19	20	21	22	22	23	24	25	25	26	27	28	29	30	31	32	32	
5'9"-175.2	14	15	16	17	17	18	19	20	20	21	22	22	23	24	25	25	26	27	28	28	29	30	31	31
5'10"-177.8	14	15	15	16	17	18	18	19	20	20	21	22	23	23	24	25	25	26	27	28	28	29	30	30
5'11"-180.3	14	14	15	16	16	17	18	18	19	20	21	21	22	23	23	24	25	25	26	27	28	28	29	30
5'12"-182.8	13	14	14	15	16	17	17	18	19	19	20	21	21	22	23	23	24	25	25	26	27	27	28	29
5'13"-185.4	13	13	14	15	15	16	17	17	18	19	19	20	21	21	22	23	23	24	25	25	26	27	27	28
5'14"-187.9	12	13	14	14	15	16	16	17	18	18	19	19	20	21	21	22	23	23	24	25	25	26	27	27
5'15"-190.5	12	13	13	14	15	15	15	16	17	18	18	19	20	20	21	21	22	22	23	24	25	25	26	26
5'16"-193.0	12	12	13	14	14	15	15	16	17	17	18	18	19	20	20	21	22	22	23	23	24	25	25	26

Illustration 3: BMI Chart

Diet Change

As mentioned earlier, make sure you don't immediately jump into changing your whole regular diet to a Paleo one. In order to achieve optimal results, you could start by changing 1 meal per week.

Exercise Routine

Make up an exercise routine which suits your busy schedule. Now obviously you don't want to go for 35+ hour's right? Start off by going for some light sprint or fast-paced walking once a week. Increase your activity. You could begin with minimal (heavy) lifting, add walking up and down a couple sets of stairs. Then increase the activity such as walking for 30 minutes two times a week.

As for the Carbohydrates part. You might go for the following table which will give you an idea of how you should balance your Carbohydrate intake.

	% Carbs	Carb(Grams) For Men	Carb(Grams) For Women	Goal/ Population
Very Low Carb	<10%	<65g	<50g	.Neurilogical Issues (Epilepsy,,Alzheimer's , etc) .Severe blood sugar problems
Low Carb	10%-15%	65-100g	50-75g	.Weight Loss .Blood Sugar Regulation .Mood Disturbances .Digestive Problems
Moderate Low Carb	15%-30%	100-200g	75-150g	.Generally Healthy .Maintain Weight .Adrenal fatigue .Hypothyroidism .Hipercholesterolemia
High Carb	>30%	>200g	>150g	.Atheltes and highly active people .Trying to gain weight/ muscle .Fast Metabolism,etc

Illustration 4: Carbohydrate Intake

Chapter 2: Delicious Breakfasts

Chocolate Chunk Banana Bread

(Prep time: 10 minutes\ Cook time: 50 minutes| 10 servings)

While it is true that Banana bread is really cool, you can't go wrong with banana bread dipped in chocolate! Simple yet elegant recipe will help you start off your day with a burst of chocolaty goodness and a healthy aura.

Ingredients:

- 4 medium Bananas, mashed
- 4 eggs
- ½ cup of almond butter
- 4 Tablespoons of melted coconut oil
- ½ cup of coconut flour
- ½ teaspoon of cinnamon
- 1 teaspoon of baking powder
- 1 teaspoon of pure vanilla extract
- Pinch of salt
- 6 ounces dark chocolate, chopped

Preparation:

Preheat oven 350F

1) Grease a 9 x 5 loaf pan.
2) In a large bowl, combine the mashed banana, coconut oil, eggs, pure vanilla extract and nut butter. Stir well.
3) Add the cinnamon, coconut flour, baking soda, sea salt and baking powder. Stir until combined.
4) Pour into greased pan.
5) Bake 40 minutes, for square pan, or 60 minutes for loaf pan.
6) Check center with a tooth pick, remove when it comes out clean.
7) Allow to cool for 30 minutes before removing from pan.

Nutrition Values

- Calories: 250
- Fat: 18.2g
- Carbohydrates: 19.4g
- Protein: 6.8g
- Dietary Fiber: 3.2g

Coconut Flour Pancakes

(Prep time: 5 minutes\ Cook time: 5 minutes| 2 servings)

Who doesn't love a healthy stack of pancakes to start the day off? With this recipe, you can have your fill.

Ingredients:

- 2 teaspoons extra virgin coconut oil
- 1 Tablespoon of raw honey
- 3 large eggs
- ¼ cup of coconut milk
- ½ teaspoon of pure vanilla extract
- ¼ cup of coconut flour
- ¼ teaspoon of tartar cream
- $\frac{1}{8}$ teaspoon of baking soda
- $\frac{1}{8}$ teaspoon of sea salt

Preparation:

Preheat oven to 350F
1) In a large bowl combine all the ingredients.
2) Grease muffin tin with coconut oil or paper liners.
3) Pour batter evenly in the tin.
4) Bake 35 minutes until golden brown.
5) Cool 15 minutes before removing.

Nutrition Values

- Calories: 65
- Fat: 4.2g
- Carbohydrates: 3.6g
- Protein: 2.5g
- Dietary Fiber: 1.1g

Sweet Potato Muffins

(Prep time: 10 minutes\ Cook time: 40 minutes| 9 servings)

Were you afraid that going all Paleo you might need to sacrifice cupcakes? Well don't fret. These muffins deliver a delicious punch and your diet won't suffer for it.

Ingredients:

- ¾ cup of mashed sweet potatoes
- ½ cup of shredded carrot
- ½ cup of grated apple
- ½ cup of shredded coconut
- ½ cup of raisins
- ¼ cup of chopped up dried figs
- ½ cup of chopped up walnuts
- ¾ cup of almond flour
- ⅛ cup of maple syrup
- 1 teaspoon of cinnamon
- ⅛ teaspoon of nutmeg
- 1 teaspoon of baking powder
- 2 eggs

Preparation:

1) In a large bowl, mix coconut oil and honey. Mix until combined. Add the eggs one at a time. Stir well.
2) Add the vanilla and coconut milk. Mix well until smooth.
3) Add the coconut flour. Mix until smooth.
4) Once combined, add tartar cream, salt, and baking soda. Mix well.
5) Heat ghee or coconut oil in frying pan on medium heat. Using a ladle, pour small portion of batter in pan. Swirl the mixture until a thin layer covers the bottom of pan.
6) Once bottom is golden brown, flip to other side. Cook until golden brown.
7) Serve hot with maple syrup.

Nutrition Values

- Calories: 100
- Fat: 5g
- Carbohydrates: 10g
- Protein: 6g
- Dietary Fiber: 5g

Blueberry Coconut French Toast

(Prep time: 15 minutes\ Cook time: 40 minutes| 8-10 servings)

This French toast is a dreamy delight for those who are looking for something a little bit sweet with bits of crunch and berry goodness.

Ingredients:

- 1 french baguette
- 2.5 cups of coconut milk
- 6 eggs
- 1 teaspoon of cinnamon

- ½ teaspoon of salt
- 1 cup of fresh blueberries
- 1 cup of unsweetened shredded coconut

For the Sauce

- 2 cups of blueberries
- ¾ cup of water

- 1 teaspoon of honey
- 1 Tablespoon of lemon juice

Preparation:

1) Grease a 9 x 13 baking dish.
2) Slice the baguette into one inch slices. Place them in a single layer in the baking dish.
3) In a separate bowl, combine the eggs, salt, milk, and cinnamon. Stir until well combined.
4) Pour mixture over slices of bread. Turn them to coat evenly.
5) Sprinkle some coconut. Marinade in the fridge overnight.
6) When ready to cook, preheat oven to 350F.
7) Add 1 cup of blueberries to the prepared French toast.
8) Bake for 40 minutes, until golden brown.
9) As the french toast cooks, in a small saucepan, combine the ingredients for the blueberry sauce.
10) Gently cook on medium, until desired consistency is achieved.
11) Once the french toast is cooked, serve on plates, pour the blueberry sauce over french toast.

Nutrition Values

- Calories: 111
- Fat: 8g
- Carbohydrates: 5g
- Protein: 5.5g
- Dietary Fiber: 3g

Breakfast Casserole

(Prep time: 10 minutes\ Cook time: 70 minutes| 6 servings)

Making a perfect casserole can be somewhat of a challenge. But this one has been carefully crafted and outlined to make sure it is successful.

Ingredients:

- 2 large sweet potatoes, washed, peeled, sliced
- ¼ onion, chopped
- 1 garlic clove, minced
- 3 Tablespoons of olive oil
- ¼ cup mushrooms, sliced
- ½ cup Italian sausage
- 10 eggs
- 1 green onion, sliced
- Salt and pepper

Preparation:

1) In a large frying pan, heat up 1 tablespoon of oil. Add the garlic and onion. Sauté until translucent.
2) Add diced sweet potatoes. Add more oil if needed. Cook for 15 minutes, until fork tender.
3) Place potatoes in a thin layer in greased baking dish.
4) Add the sliced mushrooms to the frying pan. Sauté for 2 minutes, until tender. Season with salt and pepper. Place the mushrooms in a thin layer over the potatoes.
5) Next, cook the sausage in the pan. Season with salt and pepper.
6) As the sausage cooks, preheat oven to 350F.
7) In a large bowl, whisk the eggs. Season with salt and pepper. Pour over the layers in the baking dish.
8) Bake the casserole for 70 minutes, until the eggs are no longer runny.
9) Serve hot.

Nutrition Values

- Calories: 287
- Fat: 19g
- Carbohydrates: 13g
- Protein: 16g
- Dietary Fiber: 2g

Tropical Sunrise Smoothie

(Prep time: 5 minutes\ Cook time: nil| 1 serving)

Want to maintain a strict diet and remain healthy? Don't look any further. Blend up this smoothie!

Ingredients:

Portion 1

- ½ a frozen banana
- ½ cup of fresh orange juice
- ¾ cup of frozen mango
- ¼ cup of water

Portion 2

- ½ a frozen banana
- ¾ cup of frozen strawberries
- ½ cup of water
- a few ice cubes

Preparation:

1) Blend the first portion of ingredients. Pour into a glass.
2) Quickly blend the ingredients of second portion.
3) Pour half of second portion to portion 1 mixture, mix them together
4) Once an orange pinkish texture has been achieved, very slowly pour the mixture into the cup with portion 1
5) Then add rest of portion 2 mixture. Stir slowly.
6) And you are done. Enjoy!

Nutrition Values

- Calories: 240
- Fat: 8g
- Carbohydrates: 22g
- Protein: 20g
- Dietary Fiber: 6g

Pumpkin Smoothie

(Prep time: 3 minutes\ Cook time: nil| 2 servings)

A healthy kick to your morning or afternoon. Whipping this up will give you energy to fulfill all the tasks on your 'to do' list.

Ingredients:

- ½ a ripe banana
- ½ cup of pumpkin puree
- 2 cups of almond milk
- 2 Tablespoons of peanut butter
- 5 ice cubes
- 2 dates
- $\frac{1}{8}$ teaspoon of ground ginger
- ¼ teaspoon of cinnamon
- Pinch of nutmeg

Preparation:

1) Add all the ingredients to the blender. Combine until smooth.
2) Serve cold!

Nutrition Values

Calories: 220 Fat: 6.4g Carbohydrates: 38g Protein: 5.6g Dietary Fiber: 6.1g

Crunchy Homemade Granola

(Prep time: 10 minutes\ Cook time: 40 minutes| 2 servings)

No more will you need to buy processed granola.

Ingredients:

- 2 cups of raw walnuts
- 2 cups of raw cashew
- 1 cup of raw pumpkin seeds
- ¼ cup oats
- 1 cup of unsweetened shredded coconut
- 1 cup of dried cranberries
- 1 egg white
- 2 Tablespoons of water
- 3 Tablespoons of grapeseed oil
- ⅓ cup of honey
- 1 teaspoon of pure vanilla extract
- ½ teaspoon of ground cinnamon
- ½ teaspoon of kosher salt

Preparation:

Preheat oven to 300F.
1) Line a cookie sheet with parchment paper.
2) Toss first 3 ingredients in food processor. Pulse until chopped.
3) In a large bowl, whisk egg white until fluffy, approximately 2 minutes.
4) Add grape seed oil, pure vanilla extract, honey, cinnamon and pinch of salt to egg white mixture. Whisk until combined.
5) Pour the chopped nuts and oats into the mixture. Stir until evenly coated.
6) Add the cranberries and shredded coconut to mixture. Stir well.
7) Pour the mixture in a thin layer on your cookie sheet.
8) Bake for 30 minutes, until golden brown.
9) Let it rest 10 minutes before eating.
10) Once completely cooled, store in air tight container.

Nutrition Values

- Calories: 265
- Fat: 19.1g
- Carbohydrates: 20.2g
- Protein: 7.4g
- Dietary Fiber: 3.7g

Protein Pancakes

(Prep time: 5 minutes\ Cook time: 10 minutes\ 4 servings)

Ingredients:

- 1 Tbsp vanilla whey protein
- ¼ cup almond flour
- 3 Tbsp whole grain soy flour
- 1 tsp baking powder
- 3 large sized whole eggs
- ⅓ cup cottage cheese, creamed
- Butter for Cook

Preparation:

1) In a bowl, combine almond meal, protein powder, baking powder and soy flour. Stir.
2) In a separate bowl, whisk the eggs. Add the creamed cottage cheese. Stir until combined. Add to dry ingredients. Stir until combined.
3) On a large griddle/skillet, melt butter over surface. Scoop out ¼ cup of batter. Cook 2-3 minutes per side, until golden brown.

Nutrition Values

- Calories: 191
- Fat: 9.9g
- Carbs: 4.4g
- Protein: 20g
- Dietary Fiber: 1.6g

Almond and Coconut Mug Muffin

(Prep time: 3 minutes\ Cook time: 1 minutes\ 1 serving)

Who doesn't love a filling muffin full of yummy goodness, especially if you can make it in a mug, in a minute?

Ingredients:

- 2 Tbsp almond flour
- ⅓ Tbsp Sucralose-based sweetener
- ⅓ Tbsp organic high fiber coconut flour
- ¼ tsp minced almonds
- Pinch of dried coconut
- ½ tsp Cinnamon
- ¼ tsp baking powder
- ⅛ tsp salt
- 1 large egg
- 1 tsp extra virgin olive oil

Preparation:

1. In a larger coffee mug, add the almond flour, sweetener, coconut flour, minced almond, dried coconut, cinnamon, baking powder, salt. Stir with a fork.
2. Crack in the egg. Pour in olive oil. Stir until combined.
3. Pop into the microwave. Cook for 1 minute. Cook at 15 second intervals if more time required.
4. Top with butter and more minced almond. Use a spoon to dig out the goodness.

Nutrition Values

- Calories: 207
- Fat: 16.8g
- Carbs: 3.5g
- Protein: 9.7g
- Dietary Fiber: 3g

Pineapple Smoothie

(Prep time: 5 minutes\ Cook time: 1 minutes\ 1 serving)

This pineapple smoothie will cool you down as it fills you up.

Ingredients:

- ½ cup plain yogurt
- ¼ cup fresh or frozen pineapple pieces
- 20 blanched almonds
- ½ cup almond milk

Preparation:

1. In a blender, combine yogurt, pineapple, almonds, almond milk. Blend until a smooth consistency.
2. You can add ice cubes if you want a cooler smoothie.

Nutrition Values

- Calories: 280
- Fat: 18.6g
- Carbs: 17g
- Protein: 10.8g
- Dietary Fiber: 4.2g

Apple Muffin with Pecan Streusel

(Prep time: 15 minutes\ Cook time: 25 minutes\ 8 servings)

These apple muffins are sure to be a crowd pleaser.

Ingredients:

Batter

- 1 cup almond flour
- 2 Tbsp of high fiber coconut flour, organic
- ¼ tsp salt
- 1 tsp baking powder

- 6 Tbsp granulated sugar substitute Erythritol
- Small pinch of Stevia
- ½ tsp cinnamon

- 2 large eggs
- ¼ cup unsweetened coconut milk
- 2 tsp pure vanilla extract
- 1 apple, chopped

Streusel

- ⅔ cup almond flour
- 6 tsp cinnamon
- ⅓ tsp salt

- 2 tsp Erythritol
- ½ cup chopped pecans
- Small pinch of Stevia
- 2 Tbsp melted butter

Preparation:

Preheat oven to 350F

1. In a small bowl, combine streusel ingredients; flour, cinnamon, salt, Erythritol, stevia and pecans. Pour in the melted butter. Stir with a fork until crumble mixture forms.
2. In a large bowl, mix the almond flour, coconut flour, salt, baking powder, cinnamon, Erythritol, Stevia, and cinnamon together.
3. In a separate bowl, whisk the eggs. Add the coconut milk, and vanilla extract. Stir in the apple pieces until a batter forms.
4. Prepare a muffin tin with 8 liners.
5. Fill the muffin cups 2/3 full. Top with a tablespoon of streusel.
6. Bake 25 minutes. Stick a toothpick in muffin, if it comes out dry, muffins are ready. Cool 10 minutes in tin.

Nutrition Values

- Calories: 242
- Fat: 20.6g
- Carbs: 5.3g

- Protein: 7.5g
- Dietary Fiber: 4.2g

Cinnamon Pie Crust With Fruit Filling

(Prep time: 10 minutes\ Cook time: 30 minutes\ 4-6 servings)

This is a fantastic pie crust base to build any pie on.

Ingredients:

- ¼ tsp salt
- 1 tsp Sucralose based sweetener
- 1 tsp cinnamon
- ½ cup unsalted cold butter, cubed
- 3 servings ⅓ cup all-purpose low-carb baking mix
- 2 Tbsp tap water
- 4-6 Tbsp sugar-free fruit jam (your choice)
- 1 egg, beaten

Preparation:

1. In a food processor, combine baking mix, cinnamon, sugar substitute. Pulse 30 seconds. Add the butter. Pulse again until a coarse crumble forms.
2. Pour in water as you pulse until a dough forms. Pulse for another 30 seconds until combined.
3. Once dough is formed, transfer to plastic wrap. Wrap and form into a 3-inch disk.
4. Chill for 30 minutes.
5. Dust a flat surface, roll out the dough.
6. Preheat oven to 400F.
7. Cut the dough into 6-8 squares, 3 x 3, ¼ inch thick. (This is approximate based on how large you roll out the dough.) Place the dough on parchment covered cookie sheet.
8. Add 1 tablespoon of fruit jam. Dap the edges with egg wash (egg beaten in a bowl). Place a square of dough over the bottom square of dough. Press down with a fork along the edges to close. Pierce the top of dough to allow steam to escape.
9. Bake 20 minutes, until golden brown.

Nutrition Values

- Calories: 243
- Fat: 18.6g
- Carbs: 4.5g
- Protein: 18.8g
- Dietary Fiber: 2.7g

Waffles

(Prep time: 10 minutes\ Cook time: 30 minutes\ 8 servings)

A sweet treat for the morning!

Ingredients:

- 3 servings ⅓ cup all-purpose low carb baking mix
- 2 tsp baking powder
- ¼ tsp salt
- 1 packet of sucralose based sweetener
- 1 large egg
- 1 cup half and half cream
- Butter for cooking

Preparation:

1. In a large bowl, whisk the dry ingredients; baking mix, baking powder, sugar substitute, and salt together.
2. In a separate bowl, whisk the eggs and half and half together. Pour into dry ingredients. Stir until a batter forms.
3. Let the batter rest for 5 minutes to activate the baking powder.
4. Heat up your waffle maker. Brush with butter.
5. Pour ¼ to ½ cup of batter onto heated square. Close the lid. Cook approximately 10 minutes, or instructions according to your waffle iron.
6. Top with maple syrup or fruit.

Nutrition Values

- Calories: 193
- Fat: 9g
- Carbs: 5.9g
- Protein: 21.4g
- Dietary Fiber: 1.9g

Egg filled Bell Pepper Rings

(Prep time: 10 minutes\ Cook time: 5 minutes\ 1 serving)

Bell peppers are usually spicy but with the egg, it takes off the bite for a different take on breakfast.

Ingredients:

- 1 tsp extra virgin olive oil
- ½ sweet red pepper, sliced into ½ inch rings
- 2 eggs
- ¼ cup shredded mozzarella cheese, optional
- Pinch of salt and pepper
- Fruit side: ¼ a banana, ¼ a small apple, ½ a kiwi, ¼ cup raspberries

Preparation:

1. Heat the oil in a skillet. Place the red pepper rings in. Sauté one side for 2 minutes. Flip over. Crack an egg in each ring. Season with salt and pepper.
2. Add 1-2 tablespoons of water to pan. Cover with a lid. Cook for 3-5 minutes, depending on desired texture of egg.
3. Optional: top with grated cheese, cover for 1 minute to allow the cheese to melt.
4. Serve with fruit on the side.

Nutrition Values

- Calories: 361
- Fat: 20g
- Carbs: 20.1g
- Protein: 19.9g
- Dietary Fiber: 5.8g

Baked Egg and Asparagus

(Prep time: 5 minutes\ Cook time: 10 minutes\ 1 serving)

Bake an egg over a bed of asparagus; healthy fulfilling breakfast.

Ingredients:

- 4 small spears asparagus, woodsy end chopped off
- 2 eggs
- 1 Tbsp parmesan cheese
- $\frac{1}{8}$ tsp garlic powder
- Pinch of fresh ground black pepper

Preparation:

Preheat oven to 400F

1. Grease a small oven-safe baking dish.
2. Steam the asparagus for 2 minutes.
3. Drain, rinse under cold water and pat dry.
4. Arrange the asparagus in a circle around the baking dish. Crack in 2 eggs. Season with garlic powder, pepper.
5. Bake 5 minutes. Remove from oven. Sprinkle parmesan cheese over top. Return to oven for 3 minutes.
6. Serve immediately.

Nutrition Values

- Calories: 471
- Fat: 40g
- Carbs: 5.6g
- Protein: 20.8g
- Dietary Fiber: 4g

Breakfast Tacos

(Prep time: 10 minutes\ Cook time: 15-20 minutes\ 3 servings)

Taco Tuesday for breakfast!

Ingredients:

- 1 cup shredded mozzarella cheese
- 6 eggs
- 2 Tbsp butter
- 3 strips of bacon
- ½ an avocado, thinly sliced
- ½ cup shredded cheddar cheese
- Pinch of salt and pepper

Preparation:

Preheat oven to 375F
1. Cook the bacon. Set aside.
2. You are going to make your very own cheese taco shells. Suspend a yard stick/ruler/long spoon between two items that prop it 6 inches from a counter.
3. Heat a skillet. Scoop half a cup of mozzarella cheese on the surface. Spread into a circle. Cook for 3 minutes until golden brown. Flip, cook on other side. Lift the circle of cheese off surface, drape it over yardstick/ruler. Let it cool as you cook the others and rest of ingredients.
4. In a separate bowl, whisk the eggs. Season with salt and pepper. Melt butter in a skillet. Scramble the eggs.
5. Prepare the tacos: Place a slice of bacon in cheese taco shell. Add a couple spoons of cooked egg. Top with shredded cheddar cheese and sliced avocado.

Nutrition Values

- Calories: 443
- Fat: 36.2g
- Carbs: 4.7g
- Protein: 3g
- Fiber: 1.7g
- Dietary Fiber: 25.7g

Breakfast Burger

Prep time: 5 minutes\ Cook time: 10-15 minutes\ 6 servings)

A real burger might be out of your reach but this meat packed breakfast burger won't be.

Ingredients:

- 2 cups lean ground sausage
- 1 cup shredded pepper jack cheese
- 6 slices of bacon
- 6 eggs
- 1 Tbsp of PB fit powder
- Pinch of salt and pepper

Preparation:

1. Cook the bacon, set aside.
2. In a bowl, combine the ground sausage, salt and pepper. Form palm-size patties.
3. In a separate bowl, combine PB Fit powder and 1 teaspoon of water. Stir until combined. Add a little more water for runnier consistency. Set aside.
4. Cook the sausage patties. Once cooked on both sides, cover one side with pepper jack cheese. Let it melt.
5. Cook the eggs, sunny side up or broken yolk, your preference.
6. Assemble the burgers: A sausage patty, slice of bacon, fried egg, dollop of PB fit powder. Serve immediately.

Nutrition Values:

- Calories: 655
- Fat: 56g
- Carbs: 3.5g
- Protein: 30.5g
- Fiber: 0.5g
- Net Carbs: 3g

Ham and Cheddar Omelet

(Prep time: 5 minutes\ Cook time: 20 minutes\ 5 servings)

Go for the luxury and indulge yourself with this Ham and Cheddar Chive Soufflé.

Ingredients:

- 2 ham steaks
- 1 Tbsp butter
- ½ onion, diced
- 1 garlic clove, minced
- 7 eggs

- 1 cup shredded cheddar cheese
- ½ cup heavy cream
- Pinch of salt and pepper
- 1 Tbsp freshly chives, chopped

Preparation:

Preheat oven to 400F

1. Cook the ham steak, dice into cubes.
2. In a large bowl, combine the eggs, heavy cream, salt and pepper. Whisk until combined. Add the cubed ham.
3. Using a skillet for the oven, melt the butter. Sauté onion and garlic for 2 minutes. Pour in the egg/ham mixture.
4. Bake 20 minutes, until golden brown.
5. Garnish with chopped chives.

Nutrition Values:

- Calories: 403.8
- Fats: 39.6g
- Carbs: 3.7g

- Protein: 19.6g
- Fiber: 0.2g
- Net Carbs: 3.5g

Mini Pancake Donuts

(Prep time: 5 minutes\ Cook time: 3-5 minutes \ 22 servings)

Craving a pancake and a donut? These easy to make and tasty to eat.

Ingredients:

- 6 Tbsp cream cheese
- 3 eggs
- 4 Tbsp almond flour
- 1 Tbsp coconut flour
- 1 tsp baking powder
- 1 tsp pure vanilla extract
- 4 Tbsp Erythritol
- 10 drops liquid stevia

Preparation:

1. Using a hand blender, mix the cream cheese until smooth. Add one egg at a time, Blend after each egg until fully combined.
2. In a separate bowl, combine the almond flour, coconut flour, baking powder, Erythritol. Mix well. Add the dry ingredients slowly to the cream cheese. Blend until combined. Add the vanilla, liquid stevia. Stir until a batter forms.
3. Donut maker instructions: heat canola oil. Drop in batter by tablespoon full. Cook 2 minutes, open lid, flip to other side. Cook until golden brown.
4. Donut pan instructions: grease the pan. Bake in oven at 350F for 17-20 minutes, until golden brown.
5. Cool 5 minutes.

Nutrition Values:

- Calories: 32.1
- Fat: 2.7g
- Carbs: 0.7g
- Protein: 1.4g
- Fiber: 0.3g
- Net Carbs: 0.4g

Pizza Waffles

(Prep time: 10 minutes\ Cook time: 3-5 minutes\ 2 servings)

Who doesn't love pizza! We all do. Now imagine having pizza, for breakfast.

Ingredients:

- 4 eggs
- 1 Tbsp parmesan cheese
- 3 Tbsp almond flour
- 1 Tbsp of psyllium husk powder
- 1 Tbsp bacon grease or canola oil
- 1 Tbsp baking powder
- 1 tsp italian seasoning
- 14 slices pepperoni, diced
- Pinch of salt and pepper
- ½ cup tomato sauce
- ½ cup shredded cheddar cheese

Preparation:

1. In a bowl, combine the eggs, parmesan cheese, almond flour, husk powder, bacon powder, bacon grease or oil, Italian seasoning, pepperoni, salt, and pepper. Stir until a batter forms.
2. Heat waffle maker. Lightly brush with canola oil. Pour in ¼ to ½ cup of batter. Close waffle maker. Cook 10 minutes, or until golden brown.
3. Preheat oven to broil.
4. Remove waffles. Place on baking sheet.
5. Spoon 1 tablespoon of tomato sauce over waffle. Sprinkle cheddar cheese on top.
6. Place waffles under broiler for 1-2 minutes, until cheese melts.

Nutrition Values:

- Calories: 525.5
- Fats: 41.5g
- Carbs: 10.5g
- Protein: 29g
- Fiber: 5.5g
- Net Carbs: 5.0g

Chapter 3: Mouth-Watering Lunches

Taco Salad In A Mason jar

(Prep time: 10 minutes\ Cook time: 20 minutes| 2 servings)

While usually we use mason jars to store pickles, in this recipe we are going to be using our Mason Jar to store a finely prepared Taco Salad!

Ingredients:

- 2 -3 Tablespoons olive oil
- 8 ounce chicken breast, cut into bite sized pieces
- 2 carrots, sliced
- 1 large red bell pepper, sliced
- ½ onion, roughly chopped
- 2 garlic cloves, minced
- 2 teaspoons of cumin seed
- 1 large avocado, diced
- Juice from 1 lime
- 1 cup of salsa
- 2 cups Roma tomatoes, chopped
- ½ cucumber, chopped
- ½ cup cilantro, roughly chopped
- ½ cup fresh spinach, roughly chopped
- 2 quart wide-mouth mason jars
- Pinch of salt and pepper

Preparation:

1) In a large skillet, pour in 1 tablespoon olive oil, heat it over medium.
2) Add the garlic and onion. Sauté until translucent.
3) Toss in the chicken breast, cook until golden brown.
4) Drizzle oil into pan with chicken. Add the carrots. Cook for 3 minutes.
5) Reduce heat to low, add bell pepper.
6) In a separate pan, over medium /high heat toast the cumin seeds for 2 minutes. Gently transfer them from there to a cutting board. Crush them gently. Add the seeds to the pan of chicken and vegetables.
7) Dice the avocado. Place in food processor. Pour in the lime juice. Pulse until smooth.

8) Then take your mason jar and pour ½ cup of salsa in the bottom. Pour in avocado mixture next.

9) Add the chicken and vegetables next. Add a layer of tomatoes, cucumbers, cilantro, and spinach leaves. When ready to eat, toss with your favorite paleo-friendly dressing.

Nutrition Values

- Calories: 177
- Fat: 9.1g
- Carbohydrates: 9.8g

- Protein: 16g
- Dietary Fiber: 4.7g

Lettuce Tacos with Chipotle Chicken

(Prep time: 20 minutes\ Cook time: 30 minutes| 4 servings)

If you are in the mood for chicken and something crunchy, this recipe will satisfy both cravings. The Chipotle chicken is perfect with your lettuce Tacos.

Ingredients:

- 2 large chicken breasts, sliced
- 2 – 3 Tablespoons of olive oil
- 1 red onion, finely sliced
- 2 garlic cloves, minced
- 1 small tin of diced tomatoes
- 1 teaspoon of finely chopped chipotle
- ½ teaspoon of cumin

- Pinch of brown sugar
- 8 – 10 leaves Large lettuce
- Fresh coriander leaves
- Sliced up pickled jalapeno chilies
- Slices of guacamole
- 1 tomato, sliced
- Lime wedges

Preparation:

1) In a large frying pan, drizzle oil over bottom of pan. Sauté the sliced onion and garlic until translucent.

2) Add the chicken. Cook until golden brown. Set aside.

3) Add tomatoes, brown sugar, cumin, chipotle to pan. Simmer 10 minutes, until tomato fork tender and a sauce starts to form.

4) Return chicken to the pan. Stir until chicken evenly coated. Simmer for 5 minutes.

5) Assemble rest of ingredients in bowls to make tacos.

6) Place a lettuce leaf on a plate. Top with chicken. Option to add other toppings: pickled jalapeno, guacamole, fresh tomato slice. Drizzle lime juice over ingredients.

Nutrition Values

- Calories: 332
- Fat: 15.7g
- Carbohydrates: 13.9g
- Protein: 34.3g
- Dietary Fiber: 2.1g

Spicy Picadillo Lettuce Wrap

(Prep time: 10 minutes\ Cook time: 25 minutes| 6 servings)

Yet another recipe involving Lettuce Wrap, but this time a little bit more over the top with finely crafted Paleo suitable Lettuce Tacos!

Ingredients:

For the Picadillo

- 1 pound of grass fed ground beef
- 2 Tablespoons of coconut oil
- 1 onion, diced
- 1 garlic clove, minced
- ½ teaspoon of salt
- 1 teaspoon fresh ground black pepper
- 1 teaspoon of ground cumin
- ½ teaspoon of ground cinnamon
- 1 x 14 ounce can whole tomatoes
- ¼ cup of currants
- 2 Tablespoons of green olives
- 2 Tablespoons of drained capers
- 2 Tablespoons of olive brine

For the Pico De Gallo

- ½ cup of minced red onion
- ⅔ cup of diced tomatoes
- 2 Tablespoons of minced cilantro
- 2 teaspoons of fresh lime juice
- Pinch of salt, pepper

Serving

- Large leaf lettuce
- Cooked brown rice
- Chopped cilantro

Preparation:

1) In a large frying pan, drizzle oil over bottom. Sauté onion and garlic for 1 minute. Add the ground beef. Break into small pieces. Cook until no longer pink in middle.
2) Add the bell pepper. Cook until fork tender.
3) In a separate pot, heat the canned tomatoes, currants, diced olives, olive brine, and capers. Add the cooked beef. Stir until combined. Bring to a boil, cook for 5 minutes.
4) Reduce temperature to simmer 10-20 minutes.
5) On the side, prepare the ingredients listed for pico de Gallo.
6) On a plate, place a large leaf of lettuce. Spoon on cooked beef, cooked rice. Garnish with fresh cilantro. Top with pico de Gallo.

Nutrition Values

- Calories: 178
- Fat: 7.8g
- Carbohydrates: 7.8g
- Protein: 20.5g
- Dietary Fiber: 1.5g

California Turkey, Bacon Lettuce Wrap with Basil Mayo

(Prep time: 10 minutes\ Cook time: nil| 2 servings)

Mixing up a fine lettuce wrap with the juicy goodness of bacon and basil mayo for an added oomph factor.

Ingredients:

For the Wrap

- 1 head of iceberg lettuce
- 4 slices of gluten-free deli turkey
- 3 slices of gluten-free bacon, cooked

- 1 avocado, thinly sliced
- 1 Roma tomato, thinly sliced

Serving

- ½ cup of gluten-free mayonnaise
- 6 large basil leaves, torn
- 1 teaspoon lemon juice

- 1 garlic clove, chopped
- Pinch of salt and pepper

Preparation:

1) In a food processor, combine the ingredients for basil mayo. Pulse until smooth consistency.
2) Place a large leaf of lettuce on a plate. Layer a slice of turkey, slice of bacon, slice of tomato, then a slice of avocado. Spread mayo over ingredients. Season with salt and pepper.
3) Tuck the ends in, roll the lettuce leaf over your filling, creating a burrito.
4) Slice in half. Serve chilled.

Nutrition Values

- Calories: 150
- Fat: 13.5g
- Carbohydrates: 17.5g
- Protein: 6.1g
- Dietary Fiber: 4g

Steak with Siracha Lettuce Wrap

(Prep time: 10 minutes\ Cook time: 10 minutes| 1 servings)

A proper meal cannot be complete without having a few pieces of steak with it, right? This recipe gives you that and more in the form of steak wrapped around in fresh wrap.

Ingredients:

- ½ pound of fajita seasoned steak strips (cut in ½ inch strips)
- 1 small onion, sliced
- 2 garlic cloves, diced
- 1 small bell pepper, diced
- 2 Tablespoons of siracha sauce
- 2 teaspoons of coconut aminos
- Sesame seed oil
- Green onions for garnish
- A handful of pea shoots
- 2 – 4 Large leaves of romaine lettuce

Preparation:

1) Drizzle oil along bottom of a large frying pan. Add the onion and garlic. Sauté on medium for 2 minutes until translucent.
2) Add the sliced fajita steak. Cook 2 minutes per side.
3) Add the bell pepper. Cook until fork tender.
4) Drizzle in more sesame seed oil. Add the pea shoots, coconut aminos, and Sirach sauce. Stir well.
5) Once the meat has absorbed the sauce, turn off the heat.
6) Spoon the mixture into lettuce leaves. Garnish with diced green onions. Serve hot.

Nutrition Values

- Calories: 268
- Fat: 13.5g
- Carbohydrates: 17.9g
- Protein: 1.9g
- Dietary Fiber: 19.3g

Cajun Shrimp Noodle Bowl

(Prep time: 5 minutes\ Cook time: 15 minutes| 2 servings)

Coming straight from the Mexican tables, this shrimp cajun delight might be a bit spicy, but definitely worth the effort! Easily made to satisfy your shrimp lust!

Ingredients:

For the Dish

- 3 garlic cloves, crushed
- 3 Tablespoons of grass fed butter
- 20 jumbo shrimp, deveined, tail off

For the Cajun Seasoning

- 1 teaspoon of paprika
- Dash of cayenne pepper
- ½ teaspoon of Himalayan Sea Salt
- Dash of red pepper flakes
- 1 teaspoon of garlic granules
- 1 teaspoon of onion powder

For Others

- 1 large zucchini, spiralized
- 1 red pepper, sliced
- 1 onion, thinly sliced
- 1 Tablespoon of grass fed butter

Preparation:

1) Spiralize the Zucchini.
2) In a large bowl, add the cajun seasoning. Add the shrimp. Toss until evenly coated with seasoning.
3) Heat a large frying pan on medium. Melt the butter. Add the garlic, onion, and red pepper. Sauté for 2 minutes.
4) Add the shrimp. Cook until shrimp turns pink.
5) In a separate frying pan, heat up the butter. Lightly sauté the Zucchini noodles for approximately 3 minutes – el dante.
6) Place the Zucchini noodles in a bowl. Top with garlic Cajun shrimp and vegetable mixture

Nutrition Values

- Calories: 92
- Fat: 7.6g
- Carbohydrates: 2.2g
- Protein: 4.6g
- Dietary Fiber: 0.8g

Egg Roll In A Bowl

(Prep time: 10 minutes\ Cook time: 10 minutes| 2 servings)

Looking for a quick fix to your Paleo Hunger? Serve up a plate of Paleo egg roll for a quick lunch to maintain your diet and get back to your busy life.

Ingredients:

- 1 small head of a cabbage, chopped into slices
- 1 skinless, boneless chicken breast, diced in bite-size pieces
- 2 large carrots
- 1 Tablespoon of unflavored coconut oil
- ⅓ cup of coconut aminos
- 1 Tablespoon of sesame seed oil
- 2 garlic cloves, minced
- 4 green onions, diced

Preparation:

1) In a large frying pan, heat up the coconut oil over medium-high heat.
2) Add the garlic. Sauté for 1 minute. Add the chicken. Cook until no longer pink in middle – depending on thickness, anywhere from 5 – 7 minutes.
3) Toss in the cabbage and carrots. Sauté until vegetables are fork tender. (You don't want them too soft. A bit of a crunch is good.)
4) Add the coconut aminos. Stir until the ingredients are coated. Simmer for a minute or two until sauce absorbed.
5) Serve into bowls. Garnish with diced green onions.

Nutrition Values

Calories: 463 Fat: 18.5g Carbohydrates: 27.8g Protein: 49.8g Dietary Fiber: 9.3g

Anti-Pasto Salad

(Prep time: 5 minutes\ Cook time: nil| 4 servings)

A hearty salad to fill any craving.

Ingredients:

- 1 large romaine lettuce, chopped into chunks
- ½ cup prosciutto, chopped into chunks
- ½ cup salami, chopped into cubes
- ½ cup of artichoke, chopped into chunks
- ½ cup black olives, whole
- ½ cup of hot or sweet peppers, whole
- Italian dressing as required

Preparation:

1) Add all the ingredients to a large bowl.
2) Drizzle in dressing. Toss until evenly coated.
3) Serve in bowls.

Nutrition Values

Calories: 240 Fat: 13g Carbohydrates: 19g Protein: 2g Dietary Fiber: 0g

Broiled Parmesan Tilapia

(Prep time: 5 minutes\ Cook time: 10 minutes\ 4-6 servings)

Fish isn't always the tastiest but adding a bit of parmesan kicks it up a notch.

Ingredients:

- 4–6 Tilapia fillets
- ½ cup finely grated parmesan cheese
- 3 Tbsp mayonnaise
- ¼ cup softened butter
- 2 Tbsp fresh lemon juice
- ¼ tsp dried basil
- $\frac{1}{8}$ tsp onion powder
- $\frac{1}{8}$ tsp celery salt
- ¼ tsp ground black pepper

Preparation:

Preheat oven to broil

1. Cover a baking sheet with aluminum foil.
2. In a small bowl, combine the mayonnaise, butter, lemon juice, basil, onion powder, celery salt, pepper. Stir until mixed well.
3. Place the Tilapia in a single layer on baking sheet. Cover one side of the fillets with the dressing. Place under broiler. Bake 2-4 minutes, until golden brown.
4. Pull out the pan, flip the fillets. Spread more dressing over fillets. Return to oven. Bake another 2-4 minutes, until golden.

Nutrition Values

- Calories: 224
- Fat: 12.8g
- Carbs: 0.8g
- Protein: 25.4g
- Dietary Fiber: 0.1g

Blue Cheese & Bacon Stuffed Pork Chops

(Prep time: 15 minutes\ Cook time: 20 minutes\ 2 servings)

A powerful smash flavors.

Ingredients:

- 2 butterfly pork chops (boneless)
- ¼ cup crumbled blue cheese
- 2 slices of bacon, cooked, crumbled
- 2 Tbsp fresh chives, chopped
- Pinch of garlic powder
- Pinch of fresh ground black pepper
- Fresh parsley, garnish

Preparation:

Preheat oven to 325F

1. Slice pork chops length-wise to create a pocket.
2. Grease a shallow baking dish with butter.
3. In a small bowl, combine the blue cheese, chives, and bacon. Mix well.
4. Divide mixture in half, roll loosely into balls.
5. Place a ball in the pocket of each butterflied pork chop. Close with a toothpick.
6. Season both sides of pork chops with garlic salt, and pepper.
7. Bake 20 minutes, until pork chops are cooked through. Flip pork chops halfway through cooking. (Pork internal temperature: 165F)
8. Remove from oven. Cover with foil and rest for 5 minutes (will allow the dressing inside to settle.) Garnish with fresh parsley.

Nutrition Values

- Calories: 394
- Fat: 26.3g
- Carbs: 2g
- Protein: 36g
- Dietary Fiber: 0.3g

Pan-Fried Tuna Patty

(Prep time: 15 minutes\ Cook time: 5 minutes\ 2 servings)

Everybody loves Tuna! Now you can enjoy it as a burger.

Ingredients:

- 1 can of tuna packed in water
- 1 egg
- ½ stalk of celery, chopped
- 2 Tbsp chopped walnuts
- 2 Tbsp fresh parsley, chopped
- 1 tsp fresh dill, chopped
- Pinch of salt and pepper
- 2 Tbsp mayonnaise
- 1 Tbsp butter
- ¼ cup shredded cheddar cheese

Preparation:

1. Drain the water from can of tuna.
2. In a bowl, combine tuna, egg, celery, chopped walnut, parsley, dill, salt, and pepper. Stir until fully combined. Add the mayonnaise. Stir again to mix.
3. Divide mixture in half. Form two round patties.
4. In a skillet, melt the butter. Cook the patties 2 minutes, flip to other side.
5. Sprinkle shredded cheese on cooked side. Cook patty another 2 minutes.
6. Serve immediately.

Nutrition Values

- Calories: 367
- Fat: 29.3g
- Carbs: 2.4g
- Protein: 24.2g
- Dietary Fiber: 0.8g

Crustless Quiche Lorraine

(Prep time: 10 minutes\ Cook time: 210 minutes\ 8 servings)

It might sound weird but give it a chance. This quiche may just surprise you.

Ingredients:

- 4 eggs
- 1 x 8 oz container sour cream
- 1 package frozen spinach, defrosted, drained, chopped
- 1 cup shredded cheese (mild, or sharp)
- ½ cup crumbled feta cheese

- ½ cup shredded parmesan cheese
- 1 onion, diced
- 1 tomato, diced
- ½ cup green chilies, drained, chopped
- 1 garlic clove, minced up tsp of garlic
- 1 tsp ground cumin
- 1 Tbsp paprika
- ¼ tsp cayenne pepper

Preparation:

Preheat oven to 325Fahrenheit

1. In a medium bowl, add the eggs. Beat them. Whisk in the sour cream until a smooth consistency.
2. Add the cheddar cheese, parmesan cheese, feta cheese, tomato, spinach, onion, green chilies, cumin, garlic, cayenne pepper, and paprika. Stir well.
3. Grease a pie plate. Pour in the batter. Place the pie plate on a baking sheet.
4. Bake 1 hour. Allow to set 5 minutes before slicing.

Nutrition Values

- Calories: 401
- Fat: 32.4g
- Carbs: 10.6g
- Protein: 19.3g
- Dietary Fiber: 2.5g

Asian Beef Salad

(Prep time: 6-10 hours, 20 minutes\ Cook time: 5 minutes\ 1 serving)

The Asian beef salad is perfect for Atkins diet.

Ingredients:

- 1 small garlic clove, minced
- ½ Tbsp tamari soy sauce
- ¼ Tbsp sodium/sugar-free rice wine vinegar
- ¼ tsp sesame oil
- ⅛ tsp based sweetener
- ⅛ tsp curry powder
- Pinch of ground ginger
- 4 pieces ¼ ounce beef top sirloin
- ½ Tbsp canola oil
- ¾ cup spring mixed salad greens
- 1 small red bell pepper
- ¼ cup water chestnuts, sliced
- 1 scallion, diced
- Asian dressing

Preparation:

1. In a Ziploc bag, combine minced garlic, soy sauce, rice wine vinegar, sesame oil, sugar, curry powder, ginger. Add steak to bag. Massage steak through bag to coat.
2. Place in the fridge to marinate over night.
3. The next day, remove the steak from the bag. (Discard the marinade.) Set on a plate to bring to room temperature before cooking, approximately 30 minutes.
4. Heat the oil in a skillet. Place the steak in the skillet. Cook 5-6 minutes per side.
5. Remove from pan. Let the steak rest 10 minutes before slicing.
6. In a large bowl, add the mixed salad greens, red bell pepper, water chest nuts, and scallion.
7. Slice the steak. Add to bowl. Drizzle in Asian dressing. Toss lightly. Serve.

Nutrition Values

Calories: 295   Fat: 13.3g   Carbs: 10.4g   Protein: 29.5g   Dietary Fiber: 4.1g

Almond And Parmesan Crusted Tilapia

(Prep time: 10 minutes\ Cook time: 10 minutes\ 4 servings)

Ingredients:

- 1 tsp olive oil
- 3 garlic cloves, minced
- ½ cup grated parmesan
- ¼ cup crushed almonds
- 2 Tbsp bread crumbs
- 1 tsp seafood seasoning
- ¼ tsp dried basil
- ¼ tsp ground black pepper
- ⅛ tsp celery salt
- ¼ cup buttery spread, softened
- 3 Tbsp reduced fat olive oil mayonnaise
- 2 Tbsp fresh lemon juice
- 4 tilapia fillets

Preparation:

Adjust oven rack to 6 inches from broiler. Preheat broiler

1. Line a baking dish with aluminum foil. Lightly grease the foil.
2. In a small skillet, heat olive oil. Sauté garlic for 3 minutes. Transfer to a bowl.
3. In the bowl, also add parmesan cheese, crushed almonds, bread crumbs, seafood seasoning, basil, pepper, celery salt. Whisk to combine. Stir in buttery spread and mayonnaise until combined. Add lemon juice. Stir until mixed in well.
4. Place tilapia fillets on aluminum foil covered baking dish.
5. Place under broiler. Cook 3 minutes. Flip to other side, cook another 3 minutes.
6. Remove from oven. Spread coating on 1 side. Return to broiler. Cook 3 minutes.
7. Remove from oven. Spread coating to other side. Return to broiler. Cook 3 minutes. Fish should be flaky, and coating golden brown. Serve hot

Nutrition Values

Calories: 344   Fat: 21.9g   Carbs: 6.6g   Protein: 29.3g   Dietary Fiber: 0.9g

Apricot Glazed Brisket

(Prep time: 15 minutes\ Cook time: 5 minutes\ 4 servings)

With this glazed Apricot Brisket, you will have no trouble winning the heart of everyone.

Ingredients:

- 2 Tbsp canola oil
- 4 pounds beef brisket
- 2 tsp salt
- 2 tsp paprika
- 1 tsp black pepper
- 2 large carrots, diced in chunks
- 1 large onion, diced in chunks
- 3 Tbsp sugar-free apricot

Preparation:

Preheat oven to 375F

1. Combine salt, pepper, paprika in a bowl. Stir until combined.
2. Spread over surface of brisket.
3. Drizzle oil over bottom of Dutch oven or pot for oven. Sear on all sides.
4. Once done, turn over brisket with fat side up. Add ½ a cup of water to pan.
5. Add carrots and onion to pan. Cook for 3-4 hours until the brisket is tender.
6. Remove brisket from oven. Spread apricot jelly over brisket. Return to oven.
7. Broil 6 inches from heat for 5 minutes until the apricot jam creates a crust.
8. Remove from oven. Cover in aluminum foil. Let it rest 15 minutes before slicing.
9. Transfer to platter. Place carrots and onions on platter or discard.

Nutrition Values

- Calories: 358
- Fat: 16g
- Carbs: 1.3g
- Protein: 47g
- Dietary Fiber: 0.3g

Simplified Barbeque Chicken

(Prep time: 10 minutes\ Cook time: 90 minutes\ 6 servings)

Ingredients:

- 6 bone-in chicken breast halves, skin on
- 1 Tbsp Worcestershire sauce
- 1 Tbsp hickory flavored liquid smoke
- 2 tsp chili powder
- 2 tsp ground cumin
- 2 tsp garlic powder
- 2 tsp dried thyme
- 2 tsp dried oregano
- Pinch of salt and pepper

Preparation:

Preheat oven to 375F

1. Lightly grease 9 x 13 baking dish. Place chicken in single layer.
2. In a bowl, combine the Worcestershire sauce, liquid smoke, chili powder, cumin, garlic powder, thyme, oregano, salt, and pepper.
3. Spread coating over pieces of chicken.
4. Cover with aluminum foil. Bake for 90 minutes.
5. Serve immediately.

Nutrition Values

- Calories: 330
- Fat: 14g
- Carbs: 2.6g
- Protein: 45.4g
- Dietary Fiber: 0.9g

Bacon, Avocado, Chicken Sandwich

(Prep time: 10 minutes\ Cook time: 25 minutes\ 2 servings)

Ingredients:

Cloud Bread

- 3 eggs
- ¼ cup cream of tartar

- ¼ cup cream cheese
- ¼ tsp salt
- ½ tsp garlic powder

Filling

- 1 Tbsp mayonnaise
- 1 tsp siracha
- 2 slices of bacon
- 1 chicken breast fillet
- 2 slices pepper jack cheese
- ¼ avocado, sliced

Preparation:

Preheat oven to 300F
1. Separate the eggs in to 2 different bowls.
2. Bowl with egg whites, add cream of tartar. Blend with electric mixer until fluffy.
3. Bowl with egg yolks, add cream cheese. Blend with electric mixer until smooth.
4. Slowly fold the fluffy egg whites in to egg yolk mixture.
5. Line a baking sheet with parchment paper.
6. Scoop ¼ cups of batter on baking sheet.
7. Smooth batter in to a circle. Sprinkle salt and garlic powder over clouds.
8. Bake 25 minutes.
9. While cloud bread is baking, in a skillet, cook the bacon, then the chicken. Season chicken breast with salt and pepper. Slice chicken breast after cooked.
10. Remove clouds from oven. Remove with a flipper to a flat surface.
11. Slice the avocado.
12. Combine mayonnaise and siracha sauce in a bowl. Stir until combined.
13. Spread a layer of spicy mayo on one cloud bread.
14. Place a slice of pepper jack cheese, then chicken, slice of bacon. Top with another cloud bread.

Nutrition Values:

- Calories: 361
- Fat: 28.25g
- Carbs: 4g
- Protein: 2g
- Fiber: 2g
- Net Carbs: 22g

Crispy Tofu And Bok Choy Salad

(Prep time: 6-7 hours, 20 minutes \ Cook time: 30-35 minutes\ 3 servings)

Tofu and Bok Choy to give you a hearty new take on tofu. Don't knock it 'til you try it.

Ingredients:

Oven baked tofu

- 1 cup extra firm tofu
- 1 Tbsp soy sauce
- 1 Tbsp sesame oil
- 1 Tbsp of water

- 2 garlic cloves, minced
- 1 Tbsp rice wine vinegar
- Juice from ½ a lemon

Bok Choy Salad

- 6 heads baby Bok Choy
- 1 green onion, diced
- 2 Tbsp cilantro, chopped
- 3 Tbsp coconut oil, heated in microwave and cooled

- 2 Tbsp soy sauce
- 1 Tbsp sambal olek
- 1 Tbsp natural peanut butter
- Juice from ½ a lime
- 2 drops liquid stevia

Preparation:

1. Wrap the tofu in a clean tea towel. Place a heavy pot/cast iron skillet on top. Press out moisture for 6 hours. Swap out tea towel for dry one at halfway point.
2. Once dried out, slice into cubes.
3. In a bowl, combine soy sauce, sesame oil, water, minced garlic, rice wine vinegar, lemon juice. Stir well. Pour marinade in large Ziploc bag. Add tofu cubes. Massage tofu through bag to coat. Marinate in fridge 30 minutes to 8 hours.
4. When ready to cook. Preheat oven to 350F. Place tofu on parchment covered baking sheet in a single layer. Bake 35 minutes.
5. As it bakes, in a bowl, combine the coconut oil, soy sauce, sambal olek, peanut butter, lime juice, stevia. Stir until combined.

6. Chop up the Bok Choy. Add the diced green onion, and cilantro.
7. Remove tofu from oven.
8. Add to bowl with Bok Choy salad. Drizzle dressing over ingredients. Serve.

Nutrition Values:

- Calories: 442.3
- Fat: 35.0g
- Carbs: 7.3g
- Protein: 25.0g
- Fiber: 1.7g
- Net Carbs: 5.7g

Cheese Stuffed Bacon Wrapped Hot Dogs

(Prep time: 5-10 minutes\ Cook time: 35-40 minutes\ 6 servings)

Sometimes you just really need a guilty pleasure.

Ingredients:

- 6 all beef hot dogs
- 12 slices of bacon
- 3 slices cheddar cheese, cut in half
- ½ tsp garlic powder
- ½ tsp onion powder
- Pinch of salt and pepper

Preparation:

Preheat oven to 300F
1. Slice the hot dogs down the middle. Place sliced cheese in middle.
2. Wrap bacon around the hot dog; might take 2 slices.
3. Secure with toothpick on each end.
4. Place on baking sheet lined with parchment paper.
5. Bake 35-40 minutes, until bacon crispy.

Nutrition Values:

- Calories: 379.7
- Fat: 34.5g
- Carbs: 0.3g
- Protein: 16.8g
- Fiber: 0g
- Net Carbs: 0.3g

Chicken Enchilada Soup

(Prep time: 10 minutes\ Cook time: 30-35 minutes\ 4 servings)

An enchilada in a soup. It is good. Trust me.

Ingredients:

- 3 Tbsp olive oil
- 1 onion, diced
- 2 garlic cloves, minced
- 3 stalks of celery, sliced
- 1 red bell pepper, diced
- 1 cup diced tomatoes
- 4 cups of chicken broth
- 1 package 8-ounce cream cheese
- ½ cup cooked chicken breast or thigh, shredded
- 2 tsp cumin
- 1 tsp oregano
- 1 tsp chili powder
- ½ tsp cayenne pepper
- Juice from ½ a lime
- Cilantro for garnish
- Shredded cheddar cheese, garnish

Preparation:

1. In a large skillet, heat the olive oil. Sauté the onion, garlic, red pepper, and celery for 5 minutes.
2. Add the tomatoes. Stir and cook for 3 minutes. Add the cumin, oregano, chili powder, cayenne pepper. Stir again.
3. Pour in the chicken broth and stir. Simmer for 10 minutes.
4. After 10 minutes, stir in the cream cheese. Simmer on low heat 5 minutes.
5. Add shredded cooked chicken. Stir. Simmer 5 minutes. Squeeze in the lime juice.
6. Serve in bowls. Garnish with cilantro and shredded cheese.

Nutrition Values:

- Calories: 344.8
- Fat: 31.3g
- Carbs: 7.8g
- Protein: 13.3g
- Fiber: 1.8g
- Net Carbs: 6.0g

Jalapeno Popper Mug Cake

(Prep time: 5 minutes\ Cook time: 10-15 minutes\ 1 serving)

If you have what it takes to survive the spiciness of jalapeno!

Ingredients:

- 2 Tbsp almond flour
- 1 Tbsp golden flaxseed
- ½ tsp baking powder
- Pinch of salt and pepper
- 1 slice of bacon
- ½ a jalapeno pepper
- 1 egg
- 1 Tbsp butter
- 1 Tbsp cream cheese

Preparation:

1. Cook the bacon.
2. In a mug, combine the almond flour, flaxseed, baking powder, salt, pepper, bacon, jalapeno pepper. Stir everything.
3. Beat the egg slightly. Pour into mug. Stir it in.
4. Add the butter, cream cheese. Stir.
5. Microwave for 75 seconds, on power 10.
6. Fork or spoon, eat it right out of the mug.

Nutrition Values:

- Calories: 429
- Fat: 38g
- Carbs: 8.4g
- Protein: 16.5g
- Fiber: 4.2g
- Net Carbs: 4.2g

Thai Peanut Shrimp Curry

(Prep time: 10 minutes\ Cook time: 10-20 minutes\ 2 servings)

Have a bowl of rice but nothing to go with? Cook up a batch of Thai Shrimp.

Ingredients:

- 2 Tbsp coconut oil
- 1 spring onion, diced
- 1 garlic clove, crushed
- ½ tsp turmeric
- ¼ cup broccoli florets
- 2 Tbsp green curry paste
- 1 Tbsp soy sauce
- 1 Tbsp peanut butter
- 1 tsp fish sauce
- 1 cup vegetable broth
- 1 cup coconut milk
- 3 Tbsp chopped cilantro
- ¼ tsp xanthan gum
- ½ cup cream
- 1 cup pre-cooked shrimp
- Juice from ½ a lime

Preparation:

1. In a large skillet, heat the coconut oil. Sauté the minced ginger and spring onion for 1 minute. Add the turmeric and curry paste.
2. Stir in the soy sauce, peanut butter, and fish sauce. Mix them well.
3. Pour in vegetable broth and coconut milk. Add the broccoli. Simmer 5 minutes.
4. Stir in xanthan gum and cream. Add the shrimp. Simmer 10 minutes.
5. Serve over rice. Squirt lime juice over the curry.

Nutrition Values:

- Calories: 454.5g
- Fat: 31.5g
- Carbs: 13.7g
- Protein: 27g
- Fiber: 4.8g
- Net Carbs: 8.9g

Chapter 4: Flavorful Dinners

Skillet Chicken Thighs With Butternut Squash

(Prep time: 15 minutes\ Cook time: 30 minutes| 4-6 servings)

Butternut are pretty famous for their nice flavor. If you have a skillet lying around this dish can be whipped up in no time.

Ingredients:

- ½ pound of Nitrate free bacon
- 6 boneless, skinless chicken thighs
- 2 - 3 cups of butternut squash, cubed
- Extra virgin olive oil/ coconut oil for frying
- Fresh sage, finely chopped
- Salt and pepper

Preparation:

Preheat oven to 425F

1) In a large skillet over medium-high heat, fry bacon until crispy.
2) Set bacon aside. Crumble when cooled.
3) In same skillet, using the bacon grease, sauté butternut squash for a few minutes, until el dante. Season with salt and pepper.
4) Once the squash is el dante, remove from skillet.
5) Add coconut oil to skillet (if bacon grease is low).
6) Add the chicken thighs; season with salt and pepper.
7) Cook for 10 minutes until no longer pink in middle.
8) Flip them over. Return butternut squash to skillet.
9) Place skillet in preheated oven. Bake for 12 - 15 minutes, until butternut squash is fork tender.
10) Remove skillet from oven. Top with crumbled bacon and sage. Serve hot.

Nutrition Values

- Calories: 323
- Fat: 19g
- Carbohydrates: 15g
- Protein: 12g
- Dietary Fiber: 5.2g

Sweet Potato Turkey Casserole W/Eggplant and Tomato

(Prep time: 15 minutes\ Cook time: 60 minutes| 6 servings)

People don't usually consider Eggplant to be a delicious ingredient. But mix it up with sweet potato and turkey, and you have one heck of a hearty meal with a tangy kick from the tomato.

Ingredients:

For the Casserole

- 1 pound of extra lean ground turkey
- 1 medium sweet potato, peeled, diced into small pieces
- 1 medium eggplant, sliced in ½ inch pieces
- 1 Tablespoon extra-virgin olive oil
- ½ onion, chopped
- 1 garlic clove, minced

- 1 x 15 ounce can diced tomatoes
- 1 x 8 ounce can tomato paste
- Salt and pepper to taste
- ¼ teaspoon of chili powder
- ¼ teaspoon of cumin
- ⅛ teaspoon of oregano
- ⅛ teaspoon of ground cardamom
- ½ teaspoon of tarragon flakes

For the Sauce

- 1½ Tablespoons extra-virgin olive oil
- 1 cup of unsweetened almond milk

- 1 Tablespoon of almond flour
- 1 Tablespoon of coconut flour

Preparation:

Preheat oven to 350F

1) Spray an 8x8 baking/casserole dish with non-stick cooking spray.
2) Heat a large pan over medium heat. Drizzle in olive oil. Sauté onion and garlic for 2 minutes.
3) Add the turkey. Using a wooden spoon, break up the turkey and brown the meat until no longer pink. Add the sweet potatoes.
4) Stir in tomatoes and tomato paste until ingredients evenly coated.
5) Continue cooking until sweet potato pieces are el dante.

6) In a bowl, combine chili powder, cumin, oregano, cardamom, tarragon, salt and pepper. Add eggplant. Stir until eggplant coated.

7) Place eggplant in a single layer along bottom of baking dish.

8) Top with turkey and sweet potato mix. Bake for 15 minutes.

9) In a small pot, heat up the olive oil. Add the coconut flour and almond flour. Stir for 1 – 2 minutes to cook the flour. Whisk in the almond milk slowly. Stir until fully incorporated. Bring to a boil, stirring constantly. Mixture will thicken and reduce.

10) Pull the baking dish out of oven. Pour mixture over ingredients. Return to oven. Bake another 30 minutes, until top is golden brown.

11) Remove from oven. Slice into 6 servings. Garnish with fresh tarragon.

Nutrition Values

Calories: 278 Fat: 2.6g Carbohydrates: 15g Protein: 28.5g Dietary Fiber: 28.5g

Paleo Pizza Soup

(Prep time: 5 minutes\ Cook time: 30 minutes| 6 servings)

Pizza as a soup? Surprise your guests with this unique concoction that combines the flavors of pizza and delights of your favorite soup.

Ingredients:

- 1 cup chicken sausage, sliced
- ½ cup uncured pepperoni
- 1 x 25 ounce jar marinara sauce
- 1 x 14.5 ounce can fire roasted tomatoes
- ¼ cup vegetable or beef broth, no salt added
- 1 Tablespoon any flavorless oil
- 1 onion, diced
- 2 garlic cloves, minced
- ½ cup mushrooms, sliced
- 1 x 3 ounce can sliced black olives
- 1 Tablespoon of dried oregano
- 1 teaspoon of garlic powder
- Pinch of salt and pepper

Preparation:

1) In a large saucepan, heat up the oil. Sauté the onion and garlic for 2 minutes, until translucent.
2) Add sausage, peperoni, mushrooms, olives, and tomatoes to pot. Stir well. Brown until sausage and peperoni cooked through.
3) Add marinara sauce and vegetable/or beef broth. Stir in oregano, garlic powder, salt and pepper.
4) Simmer on low-medium heat approximately 30 minutes, until mushrooms are tender.
5) Serve hot

Nutrition Values

- Calories: 90
- Fat: 2g
- Carbohydrates: 17g
- Protein: 3g
- Dietary Fiber: 3g

Spicy Pumpkin Chili

(Prep time: 10 minutes\ Cook time: 15 minutes| 5 servings)

This recipe will give you the perfect blend of pumpkin with just the right amount of spicy goodness to satisfy the dragon in you.

Ingredients:

- 1 Tablespoon flavorless oil
- 2 yellow onions, chopped
- 8 garlic cloves, chopped
- 1 pound of lean ground turkey
- 2 x 15 ounce cans fire roasted tomatoes
- 2 cups of pumpkin puree
- 1 cup of chicken broth
- 2 Tablespoons of honey
- 4 teaspoons of chili spice
- 1 teaspoon of ground cinnamon
- 1 teaspoon of sea salt

Preparation:

1) In a large pot, heat the oil. Sauté onion and garlic for 2-4 minutes.
2) Add ground turkey. Using a wooden spoon, break up into small pieces. Cook until no longer pink.
3) Add the tomatoes and pumpkin puree to pot. Stir well.
4) Stir in the honey, chili spice, cinnamon, sea salt, and chicken broth. Simmer 15 minutes without a lid.
5) Serve in bowls.

Nutrition Values

- Calories: 312
- Fat: 16.2g
- Carbohydrates: 13.5g
- Protein: 27.4g
- Dietary Fiber: 27.4g

Creamy Basil And Tomato Chicken

(Prep time: 10 minutes\ Cook time: 20 minutes| 4 servings)

This recipe will give you the perfect meal if you are looking for something a little bit tangy, but has the benefits of green vegetables and protein punch of chicken.

Ingredients:

- 1 pound boneless, skinless chicken breast, diced
- ½ yellow onion
- 1 teaspoon of coconut oil
- 3 garlic cloves
- 2 Tablespoons of sunflower seeds
- 1 Tablespoon of nutritional yeast
- 1 package of fresh basil
- 1 Tablespoon of avocado oil
- Salt and pepper to taste
- ½ cup of coconut milk
- ½ teaspoon of arrowroot powder
- ⅓ cup of cold water
- 1 cup cherry tomatoes, sliced

Preparation:

1) In a large skillet, heat up the coconut oil. Add the onion and garlic. Cook for 2 minutes, until translucent.
2) Add the chicken. Cook for 12 minutes, flipping at the halfway point.
3) In the meantime, take a plate and toss in the garlic in a food processor bowl to finely mince it using the processor
4) Pour in the sunflower seeds. Pulse again, until sand-like consistency.
5) Add the nutritional yeast, salt, and pepper. Pulse until fully minced.
6) In a medium bowl, whisk the arrowroot powder with a few drops of water, to create a paste.
7) Pour in the coconut milk. Whisk until combined.
8) Pour sauce into the skillet. Stir well. Bring to a simmer.
9) Add in the sliced cherry tomatoes. Simmer 1-2 minutes. Serve hot.

Nutrition Values

Calories: 408   Fat: 31g   Carbohydrates: 9g   Protein: 23g   Dietary Fiber: 3g

Amazing Ground Turkey and Spinach Stuffed Mushroom

(Prep time: 10 minutes\ Cook time: 15 minutes| 2 servings)

Ground turkey stuffed in portobello mushrooms creates something truly delicious that is both meaty and healthy with the power of Popeye's Spinach.

Ingredients:

- 2 teaspoons of coconut oil
- 6 large Portobello mushrooms, caps cleared and gills removed.
- 1 small onion, diced
- ½ pound of lean ground turkey
- Handful of baby spinach leaves
- 6-8 grape tomatoes, sliced
- Salt and pepper to taste

Preparation:

1) In a large skillet, heat up 1 teaspoon of coconut oil. Heat the mushroom caps 2 minutes per side, until soft. Set aside.
2) Drizzle more oil in skillet. Sauté onion on medium heat for 2 minutes.
3) In the same skillet, add the ground turkey to the pan, break it up into small pieces. Cook until no longer pink. Season with salt and pepper.
4) Once cooked, remove the meat. Place tomato slices and spinach in the skillet. Heat until tomatoes soft and spinach wilted. Return meat to the pan. Stir until combined.
5) Using a spoon, scoop filling into the mushroom caps. Serve hot.

Nutrition Values

- Calories: 220
- Fat: 46g
- Carbohydrates: 14g
- Protein: 25g
- Dietary Fiber: 5g

Shepherd's Pie with Cauliflower Topping

(Prep time: 30 minutes\ Cook time: 30 minutes| 4-6 servings)

Ingredients:

- 1 head of cauliflower, chopped into florets
- 4 Tablespoons of ghee
- 1 small onion, diced
- 2 stalks of celery, diced
- 2 garlic cloves, minced
- 1 pound of lean ground beef
- ¼ - 1/2 cup of homemade beef broth
- 1 Tablespoon of homemade ketchup
- 2 Tablespoons of fresh parsley, rough chopped
- Salt and pepper to taste
- ½ - ¾ cup shredded cheddar cheese

Preparation:

Preheat oven to 400

1) Grease an 8-inch square casserole/baking dish.
2) In a large pot, steam the cauliflower until tender.
3) In a large skillet, heat up 1 tablespoon of ghee.
4) Add the onion, garlic, celery, garlic, and carrot to the skillet. Cook for 5 minutes, until vegetables are tender.
5) Add the ground beef. Brown until no longer pink. Add beef broth a bit at a time, so the meat remains wet but not saturated.
6) Add the ketchup. Season with salt and pepper. Simmer as you prepare the cauliflower.Place the cauliflower in a blender. Pulse until it is smooth. Pour in 1 tablespoon of ghee. Pulse again. Season with salt and pepper. Add parsley. Stir well.
7) Assembling: Spread a layer of meat mixture along bottom of baking dish. Top with cauliflower mix. Smooth out surface with a spoon. Cover with shredded cheddar cheese.
8) Bake 30 minutes, until cheese is melted and golden brown.

Nutrition Values

- Calories: 487
- Fat: 37g
- Carbohydrates: 11g
- Protein: 28g
- Dietary Fiber: 3.5g

Sweet and Sour Pork Chop

(Prep time: 5 minutes\ Cook time: 10 minutes| 4 servings)

Ingredients:

For the recipe

- 4 pork chops, bone in
- 1 teaspoon of fine grain salt
- $\frac{1}{8}$ teaspoon of fresh ground black pepper
- 2 Tablespoons of butter

For the glaze

- 2 Tablespoons of balsamic vinegar
- 2 Tablespoons of honey
- 2 garlic cloves, minced
- ½ teaspoon of dried rosemary
- ½ teaspoon of dried oregano
- Pinch of red pepper flakes

Preparation:

Preheat oven to 400F

1) Place a rack in the middle section.
2) Season the pork chops with salt and pepper. Set aside.
3) In a large iron skillet, melt the butter over medium-high heat.
4) While butter is sizzling, place the pork chops in the pan. Sear on both sides to create a crust. (Two minutes per side.)
5) Place the skillet in the oven, roast for 6 minutes.
6) As the meat cooks in the oven, in a saucepan, heat the balsamic vinegar, honey, garlic cloves, rosemary, oregano, red pepper flakes. Bring to a boil. Simmer to a thicker consistency.
7) Remove the skillet from the oven. Pour the sauce over the pork chops.
8) Return to the oven. Bake for 5 minutes.
9) Serve hot.

Nutr

ition Values

- Calories: 215
- Fat: 13g
- Carbohydrates: 11g
- Protein: 13g
- Dietary Fiber: 5g

Baked Lemon Pork Chops

(Prep time: 15 minutes\ Cook time: 40 minutes\ 4 servings)

Make something which the whole family can enjoy.

Ingredients:

- 4 center cut pork chops, bone in
- 8 Tbsp tamari soy sauce
- 2 Tbsp Worcestershire sauce
- 2 garlic cloves, minced
- Juice from 1 lemon, Rind from half the lemon.
- 1 tsp canola oil
- ½ tsp fresh ground black pepper

Preparation:

1. In a small bowl, combine soy sauce, Worcestershire sauce, garlic, lemon juice, lemon rind, oil, and pepper. Whisk briskly to combine.
2. Pour mixture into a large Ziploc. Add pork chops. Massage marinade into chops. Chill 1-2 hours in the fridge.
3. Preheat oven to 375F.
4. Remove pork chops from baggie. Place in a deep baking dish.
5. Bake 15 minutes. Flip over. Bake another 20 minutes.
6. Let them rest 5 minutes before serving.

Nutrition Values

- Calories: 149
- Fat: 8
- Carbs: 4g
- Protein: 15.2g
- Dietary Fiber: 0.1g

Cali Mac & Cheese

(Prep time: 15 minutes\ Cook time: 20 minutes\ 6 servings)

This recipe is designed to save you from the horror of giving up mac and cheese.

Ingredients:

- 1 large cauliflower head
- 1 cup heavy cream
- 2 Tbsp cream cheese
- 1½ tsp yellow mustard
- 1½ cups shredded cheddar cheese + cheese for top
- 1 garlic clove, minced
- Pinch of salt and white pepper
- ¼ tsp original pepper sauce

Preparation:

Preheat oven to 375F

1. Break cauliflower into small pieces (medium shell pasta size). Cook until el dante.
2. Once cooked, drain water and pat the cauliflower dry.
3. In a medium sauce pan, heat the cream to a simmer.
4. Whisk in the cream cheese. Stir in mustard until combined.
5. Add shredded cheese, salt, white pepper, garlic. Stir until cheese melted.
6. Turn the heat off. Stir in the cauliflower pieces.
7. Pour mixture into deep baking dish. Top with grated cheese.
8. Bake 15 minutes, until cheese melted and golden brown.

Nutrition Values

- Calories: 320
- Fat: 27
- Carbs: 5.6g
- Protein: 11.4g
- Dietary Fiber: 3.6g

Avocado and Cheddar Omelet

(Prep time: 15 minutes\ Cook time: 20 minutes\ 6 servings)

Care to end your day the way you started it. Breakfast for dinner?

Ingredients:

- 1 tsp canola oil
- 4 large eggs
- ½ cup shredded cheddar cheese
- 1 avocado, sliced
- ½ cup salsa
- Pinch of salt and pepper

Preparation:

1. In a large bowl, add the eggs. Whisk them to combine. Stir in salt and pepper.
2. Heat oil in a large skillet.
3. Pour in egg mixture. Cook on one side. Flip to cook other side.
4. Spread cheese and avocado on one side. Flip in half.
5. Cook 1 minute to allow cheese to melt.
6. Top with salsa. Serve hot.

Nutrition Values

- Calories: 419
- Fat: 33.6g
- Carbs: 5.2g
- Protein: 20.8g
- Dietary Fiber: 5g

Yorkshire Pudding

(Prep time: 5 minutes\ Cook time: 35 minutes\ 8 servings)

Try this pudding straight out of Yorkshire.

Ingredients:

- 3 large eggs
- 1 cup whole milk
- ½ cup whole grain soy flour
- 1 Tbsp vital wheat gluten
- 1 tsp baking powder
- Pinch of salt
- ⅓ cup canola oil

Preparation:

Pre-heat oven to 450F

1. In a bowl, whisk the eggs and milk until combined.
2. In a separate bowl, combine the soy flour, wheat gluten, baking powder, and salt. Whisk.
3. Add dry ingredients to wet ingredients. Stir until smooth.
4. Grease an 8-inch square baking dish with oil.
5. Preheat baking dish 5 minutes in oven. Once oil is smoking, remove. Pour in batter. Bake 15 minutes.
6. Reduce temperature to 350F. Bake another 15 minutes, until golden brown.
7. Serve hot.

Nutrition Values

- Calories: 157
- Fat: 11.8g
- Carbs: 3.8g
- Protein: 9.2g
- Dietary Fiber: 0.5g

Stuffed Red Bell Peppers

(Prep time: 10 minutes\ Cook time: 45 minutes\ 4 servings)

Stuffed peppers are a meal all on their own.

Ingredients:

- 2 medium sweet red peppers
- ¼ cup feta cheese
- 8 cherry tomatoes
- ½ tsp ground thyme
- 2 Tbsp basil
- 2 Tbsp extra virgin olive oil

Preparation:

Preheat oven to 400F

1. Slice the tops off the peppers. Dice the good part. Remove seeds and ribs.
2. In a bowl, combine the tomatoes, feta cheese, thyme, basil, salt, and pepper. Drizzle in 1 tablespoon of the olive oil. Stir to coat ingredients.
3. Fill pepper shells with mixture.
4. Drizzle olive oil over deep glass baking dish.
5. Place peppers in, standing up. Cover with aluminum foil.
6. Bake 30 minutes. Remove foil. Bake another 15 minutes.

Nutrition Values

- Calories: 97
- Fat: 6.8g
- Carbs: 4.6g
- Protein: 3.2g
- Dietary Fiber: 1.9g

Braised Leeks and Fennel

(Prep time: 15 minutes\ Cook time: 45 minutes\ 8 servings)

Leeks and fennel on their own are fine. Braised with chicken broth and you have a meal!

Ingredients:

- 4 leeks, diced
- 1 fennel bulb, diced
- 1 cup chicken broth
- Pinch pepper
- 3 Tbsp unsalted butter
- 1 Tbsp fresh lemon juice
- ⅓ cup parsley, chopped

Preparation:

Preheat oven to 450F

1. In an 11 x 9 glass baking dish, add the leeks, fennel. Pour in the chicken broth. Season with pepper.
2. Cut up butter. Place over the ingredients. Cover baking dish with aluminum foil.
3. Bake 15 minutes. Remove from oven.
4. Stir in lemon juice. Garnish with parsley. Serve.

Nutrition Values

- Calories: 77
- Fat: 4.6g
- Carbs: 7.1g
- Protein: 1.3g
- Dietary Fiber: 1.8g

Maple and Sage Pumpkin

(Prep time: 10 minutes\ Cook time: 15 minutes\ 8 servings)

Pumpkins naturally taste pretty good, add some maple and sage and you have created an irresistible delight.

Ingredients:

- 1 pound of pumpkin
- ¼ cup shallots, chopped
- 1 Tbsp unsalted butter
- ¼ cup vegetable broth
- ½ cup sugar-free maple syrup
- ¼ tsp ground sage

Preparation:

1. Cube the pumpkin into ¾-inch pieces.
2. In a large skillet, melt the butter. Sauté shallots and pumpkin a few minutes.
3. Season with salt and pepper.
4. Sauté 8-10 minutes, until pumpkin is tender and slightly browned.
5. Pour in maple syrup. Add sage. Stir to coat pieces. Simmer 1 minute.
6. Serve hot.

Nutrition Values

- Calories: 26
- Fat: 1.2g
- Carbs: 3.5g
- Protein: 0.6g
- Dietary Fiber: 0.4g

Spicy Buffalo Cauliflower

(Prep time: 10 minutes\ Cook time: 45 minutes\ 4 servings)

A classic way eating your vegetables. Hide it with another flavor.

Ingredients:

- 1 large head of cauliflower
- 2 Tbsp light olive oil
- Pinch of salt and pepper
- 4 Tbsp buffalo wings sauce
- 3 tsp siracha sauce
- 2 Tbsp unsalted butter
- ½ cup crumbled blue cheese

Preparation:

Preheat oven to 375F

1. Line a baking sheet with parchment paper.
2. Cut the cauliflower into small florets.
3. Drizzle 1 tablespoon of the olive oil over the florets. Season with salt and pepper.
4. Spread the florets in a single layer on the baking sheet.
5. Bake 35-40 minutes.
6. As the cauliflower bakes, in a small saucepan combine the siracha and buffalo wings sauces together. Simmer 10 minutes.
7. Stir in the butter. Pull off the heat. Allow to cool to room temperature.
8. Once cauliflower cooked, toss them with the sauce. Pour onto serving platter. Garnish with crumbled blue cheese.

Nutrition Values

- Calories: 177
- Fat: 14.9g
- Carbs: 4.1g
- Protein: 5.3g
- Dietary Fiber: 4.2g

Asian Short Ribs

(Prep time: 45-60 minutes\ Cook time: 5-10 minutes\ 4 servings)

These might not be the BBQ ribs you are accustomed to, but give them a try and you won't be disappointed.

Ingredients:

Ribs and Marinade

- 6 large short ribs
- ¼ cup soy sauce
- 2 Tbsp rice wine vinegar
- 2 Tbsp fish sauce

Spice Rub

- 1 tsp ground ginger
- ½ tsp onion powder
- ½ tsp minced garlic
- ½ tsp red pepper flakes
- ½ tsp sesame seeds
- ¼ tsp cardamom
- 1 Tbsp salt

Preparation:

1. In a small saucepan, combine rice wine vinegar, soy sauce, and fish sauce. Simmer 5 minutes. Let it cool to room temperature.
2. Pour the marinade in a large Ziploc. Place ribs in the bag. Massage marinade into ribs. Let them rest for 60 minutes.
3. In a small bowl, combine ingredients of spice rub. Dump out marinade from the Ziploc. Place ribs in a large casserole dish. Coat ribs with spice rub.
4. Fire up your grill. Cook the ribs 3-5 minutes per side.
5. Serve hot.

Nutri

tion Values:

- Calories: 416.8
- Fat: 31.8g
- Carbs: 0.9g
- Protein: 29.5g
- Fiber: 0.0g
- Net Carbs: 0.9g

Italian Stuffed Meatballs

(Prep time: 10 minutes\ Cook time: 20 minutes\ 4 servings)

They might not look fancy but they taste divine.

Ingredients:

- 1½ pounds lean ground beef
- 1 tsp oregano
- ½ tsp Italian seasoning
- 2 garlic cloves, minced
- ½ tsp onion powder
- 3 Tbsp flaxseed meal
- Pinch of salt and pepper
- 3 Tbsp tomato paste
- 1 egg
- ½ cup green olives, sliced
- ½ cup mozzarella cheese, shredded
- 1 tsp Worcestershire sauce

Preparation:

Preheat oven to 400F

1. Line a baking sheet with aluminum foil.
2. In a large bowl, combine the ground beef, oregano, Italian seasoning, onion powder, salt, and pepper. Use your hands to blend the ingredients.
3. To that mixture, add tomato paste, egg, Worcestershire and flaxseed. Mix again.
4. Slice the green olives. Shred the cheese. Combine in a bowl together.
5. Take a pinch of ground beef mixture, flatten in your palm. Place a pinch of cheese and olives mixture in the middle. Wrap ground beef around it, form a ball. Makes approximately 20-30 meatballs, depending on size. If they are on the larger size, add a bit of cooking time.
6. Place meatballs on baking sheet, 1-inch apart. Bake 20 minutes.
7. Serve hot.

Nutrition Values:

- Calories: 593.5
- Fat: 44.8g
- Carbs: 6.0g
- Protein: 36.8g
- Fiber: 2.3g
- Net Carbs: 3.8g

Nacho Chicken Casserole

(Prep time: 10 minutes\ Cook time: 20 minutes\ 6 servings)

A unique South Western variation of Shepherd's Pie.

Ingredients:

- 2 Tbsp olive oil
- 2 pounds chicken thighs, boneless, skinless
- 1½ tsp chili seasoning
- ¼ cup cream cheese
- ¾ cup cheddar cheese x 2 (one for chicken mix, one for cauliflower mix)
- 1 cup green chilies and tomatoes
- ¼ cup sour cream
- 1 cup frozen cauliflower
- 1 jalapeno pepper, diced
- Pinch of salt and pepper

Preparation:

Preheat oven to 375F

1. Cut the chicken thighs in chunk-sized pieces.
2. In a skillet, heat the oil. Sauté the chicken until golden brown. Season with salt and pepper. Stir in the sour cream, cream cheese, cheddar cheese until melted. Add the green chilies and tomatoes, and jalapeno pepper. Stir well.
3. Cook the cauliflower. Using a blender, pulse the cauliflower until a mashed consistency. Add the shredded cheese. Stir well.
4. In a deep casserole dish, pour in a layer of the chicken mixture. Add the mashed cauliflower on top. Sprinkle with jalapeno peppers.
5. Bake 20 minutes. Remove from oven. Allow to set 5 minutes before slicing.
6. Garnish with fresh cilantro.

Nutrition Values:

- Calories: 426.0
- Fat: 32.2g
- Carbs: 5.9g
- Protein: 30.8gg
- Fiber: 1.7g
- Net Carbs: 4.3g

Oven Baked Turkey Leg

(Prep time: 10 minutes\ Cook time: 20 minutes\ 4 servings)

Just because it is not Thanksgiving does not mean you can't have turkey.

Ingredients:

- 2 medium turkey legs
- 2 Tbsp duck fat
- 2 tsp salt
- ½ tsp pepper
- ¼ tsp cayenne pepper
- ½ tsp onion powder
- ½ tsp dried thyme
- ½ tsp ancho chili powder
- 1 tsp liquid smoke
- 1 tsp Worcestershire sauce

Preparation:

Preheat the oven to 350F

1. Rinse the turkey legs with water, pat them dry.
2. In a small bowl, combine the liquid smoke, Worcestershire sauce. Stir.
3. In a separate bowl, combine the salt, pepper, cayenne pepper, onion powder, thyme, chili powder.
4. In a large skillet for the oven, melt the duck fat. Sear the turkey legs on all sides.
5. Place skillet in the oven. Bake 60-70 minutes. (Turkey leg internal temp: 180F)
6. Let turkey rest 5 minutes before serving.

Nutrition Values:

- Calories: 382
- Fat: 22.5g
- Carbs: 0.8g
- Protein: 44g
- Fiber: 0g
- Net Carbs: 0.8g

Slow Cooker Braised Oxtail

(Prep time: 15 minutes\ Cook time: 6-7 hours\ 3 servings)

Oxtails are extremely juice and tempting meals.

Ingredients:

- 1 Tbsp canola oil
- 2 pounds of Oxtail, bone in
- 2 cups beef broth
- ⅓ cup butter
- 2 Tbsp soy sauce
- 1 Tbsp fish sauce
- 3 Tbsp tomato paste
- 1 tsp onion powder
- 1 tsp minced garlic
- ½ tsp ground ginger
- 1 tsp dried thyme
- Pinch of salt and pepper
- ½ tsp guar gum

Preparation:

1. In a slow cooker, heat the beef broth, fish sauce, soy sauce, butter and tomato paste.
2. In a small bowl, combine the onion powder, ginger, thyme, salt, pepper. Coat the oxtail in seasoning.
3. In a skillet, on the stove, heat up the oil. Sear the oxtail on all sides. Transfer oxtail to slow cooker. Spoon the sauce over the oxtail. Cover.
4. Cook on low 6-7 hours. Check every hour to spoon the sauce over the oxtail.
5. Once cooked, remove the oxtail to rest. Turn up the heat on the slow cooker. Stir in guar gum to thicken the sauce.
6. Set the oxtail on a platter. Cover with the sauce. Serve.

Nutrition Values:

- Calories: 433.3
- Fat: 29.7g
- Carbs: 4.2g
- Protein: 28.3g
- Fiber: 1.0g
- Net Carbs: 3.2g

Sushi

(Prep time: 10 minutes\ Cook time: 10 minutes\ 3 servings)

A sushi carved out of cauliflower and cheese.

Ingredients:

- 1 cup cauliflower florets
- 1 package, 8 oz cream cheese, room temperature
- 1-2 Tbsp rice wine vinegar
- 1-2 Tbsp soy sauce
- 6 sheets of Nori
- 1 cucumber
- ½ an avocado
- 6 thin slices smoked salmon

Preparation:

1. Place the cauliflower in a blender. Pulse until rice-like consistency.
2. Slice the avocado thinly. Peel the cucumber. Cut in spears, removing middle. Place vegetables in fridge.
3. In a skillet, heat some oil. Sauté the cauliflower rice for 5 minutes. Stir in soy sauce. Set aside to cool down.
4. In a bowl, stir the cream cheese until smooth. Slowly stir in the rice wine vinegar until combined. Place in the fridge.
5. Cover a bamboo roller with saran wrap. Place a nori sheet on bamboo roller.
6. Spread cauliflower rice mixture over sheet. Add a piece of smoked salmon on top. Add a slice of avocado and a cucumber spear. Roll up the nori sheet. Continue making rolls until ingredients used.
7. Place in fridge until ready to eat.

Nutrition Values:

- Calories: 353.3
- Fat: 25.7g
-
- Carbs: 13.7g
- Protein: 18.3g
- Fiber: 8.0g
- Net Carbs: 5.7g

Walnut Crusted Salmon

(Prep time: 10 minutes\ Cook time: 15-20 minutes\ 2 servings)

A bite of this walnut-coated salmon is a bit of heaven.

Ingredients:

- ½ cup walnuts
- 2 Tbsp sugar-free maple syrup
- ½ Tbsp Dijon mustard
- ¼ cup fresh dill
- 2 x 3 oz salmon fillets
- 1 Tbsp olive oil
- Pinch of salt and pepper

Preparation:

Preheat oven to 350F
1. Place walnuts in blender. Pulse until crumbled.
2. Chop the dill. Transfer dill and walnuts to a bowl. Pour in the maple syrup. Stir in the Dijon mustard. Whisk the ingredients until combined.
3. Coat both sides of the salmon with the mixture.
4. In a large oven skillet, heat the olive oil. Sear salmon fillets per side for 3 minutes.
5. Transfer pan to oven. Bake 8-10 minutes. Serve hot.

Nutrition Values:

- Calories: 373
- Fat: 43g
- Carbs: 4g
- Protein: 20g
- Fiber: 1g
- Net Carbs: 3g

Chapter 5: Gratifying Desserts

Graham Crackers

(Prep time: 15 minutes\ Cook time: 30 minutes| 4-6 servings)

Sometimes you feel like a snack, sometimes you don't. This graham cracker cookie can fulfill you until a next meal, and they are perfect for Paleo Diet.

Ingredients:

- 2¼ cups full almond flour
- 1 teaspoon of baking powder
- 1 teaspoon of ground cinnamon
- ½ teaspoon of fine sea salt
- 1 large egg
- 2 Tablespoons of melted coconut oil
- 2 Tablespoons of pure maple syrup

Preparation:

1) In a large bowl, whisk the dry ingredients together; almond flour, baking powder, cinnamon, and sea salt.
2) In a separate bowl, combine the egg, maple syrup, and coconut oil together. Stir until blended.
3) Pour the wet mixture into the dry ingredients. Stir until a dough forms and pulls away from the sides.
4) Cover with plastic wrap. Chill the dough for 30 minutes.
5) Preheat oven to temperature 325F. Cover a large cookie sheet with parchment paper.
6) Roll out the dough to $\frac{1}{8}$ inch thickness.
7) Using a pizza cutter or sharp knife, cut out 2.5 inch squares, transfer to cookie sheet.
8) Bake 15 minutes, until golden brown.
9) Cool 5 minutes before removing from cookie sheet.

Mango Chia Seed Pudding

(Prep time: 10 minutes\ Cook time: 60 minutes| 4 servings)

This double layer pudding will satisfy any hunger.

Ingredients:

- 3 Tablespoons of chia seeds
- 1 cup of vanilla coconut milk or almond milk
- 2 Tablespoons maple syrup
- Pinch of cinnamon
- Pinch of cardamom
- 1 teaspoon pure vanilla extract
- 1 mango, peeled, pureed

Preparation:

1) In a medium bowl with an air tight lid, combine the chia seeds, milk (coconut or almond), 1 tablespoon of the maple syrup, cinnamon, and cardamom.
2) Whisk the ingredients until combined. Place air tight lid on mixture. Refrigerate 8 – 12 hours.
3) When ready to serve. Prepare the mango: puree the mango in a food processor. Pour into a bowl. Add 1 tablespoon of maple syrup. Stir until combined. You could chill it briefly.
4) Using clear jars, alternate layers of chia pudding and mango puree. Serve immediately or refrigerate until ready to eat.

Nutrition Values

- Calories: 146
- Fat: 26g
- Carbohydrates: 15g
- Protein: 23g
- Dietary Fiber: 11.2g

Chocolaty Cocoa Mousse

(Prep time: 10 minutes\ Cook time: nil| 4 servings)

In just a few minutes, you can whip up a batch of this fine mousse.

Ingredients:

- Coconut cream scraped from upper side of 2 x 13.5 ounce cans chilled of full fat coconut milk
- 4 Tablespoons of cocoa
- 3 Tablespoons of honey
- 1 teaspoon of pure vanilla extract

Preparation:

1) The first step is to open the chilled cans of coconut milk and scoop out the thick cream. Place in a large bowl.
2) To that bowl, add the honey, cocoa, pure vanilla extract. Beat using your mixer, start low to medium until a nice foam appears.
3) Divide the mixture evenly into ramekins. Chill 30 to 60 minutes.

Nutrition Values

Calories: 134 Fat: 3.8g Carbohydrates: 16g Protein: 3.8g Dietary Fiber: 8.1g

Pumpkin Nut Butter Cup

(Prep time: 120 minutes\ Cook time: nil| 4 servings)

Who says muffins are banned on Paleo? This recipe will allow you to create exquisitely delicious pumpkin nut butter cups with multiple layers of goodness.

Ingredients:

For Filing

- ½ cup of organic pumpkin puree
- ½ cup of homemade almond butter

- 2 Tablespoons of organic maple syrup
- 4 Tablespoons of organic coconut oil
- ¼ teaspoon of organic ground nutmeg
- ¼ teaspoon of organic ground ginger
- 1 teaspoon of organic ground cinnamon
- ⅛ teaspoon of organic ground clove
- 2 teaspoons of pure vanilla extract

For Topping

- 1 cup of organic raw cacao powder
- 4 Tablespoons of organic maple syrup
- 1 cup of organic coconut oil

Preparation:

1) In a large mixing bowl, combine the pumpkin puree, almond butter, maple syrup, nutmeg, ginger, cinnamon, cloves, and vanilla extract. Blend on low to medium until smooth and creamy.
2) In another bowl, combine the cacao powder, maple syrup, coconut oil. Blend from low to medium until smooth and creamy.
3) Fill a muffin tin with paper liners. Fill the liners ⅓ full with chocolate filling. Place in freezer for 15 minutes.
4) Pour a layer ⅓ with pumpkin filling. Return to freezer for 15 minutes.
5) Pour top layer ⅓ of chocolate mix. Place in freezer. Chill for 2 hours.

Nutrition Values

- Calories: 105
- Fat: 10.1g
- Carbohydrates: 3.3g
- Protein: 2.9g
- Dietary Fiber: 1.3g

Chocolate Silk Pie

(Prep time: 90 minutes\ Cook time: 10 minutes| 16 servings)

Ingredients:

Crust:

- 28 Chocolate cookie wafers
- 2 Tablespoons sugar
- 4 Tablespoons unsalted butter, melted
- Pinch of salt

Filling:

- 8 ounces of Dark Chocolate
- ¼ cup of extra virgin olive oil
- 2 ripe Avocados
- 1 cup of coconut sugar
- 1½ cups of cocoa powder
- 1 cup of heavy cream
- 1 Tablespoon of vanilla
- ½ teaspoon of espresso powder
- Pinch of salt

Preparation:

Crust:

Preheat oven to 350F

1) Pulse the wafers, sugar, salt in food processor until you have a crumbly, sandy mixture. Add melted butter. Pulse lightly to combine.
2) Pour into a 9-inch pie pan. Press firmly on crumb mixture along bottom and up sides of pie dish.
3) Bake for 10 minutes. Allow to cool completely before filling.

Filling:

1) Melt the dark chocolate; using double-boiler method or microwave. Stir in coconut oil. Set aside. Cool to room temperature.
2) Scoop out avocado meat. Place in a mixing bowl. Mash the avocado completely until smooth.
3) Add the chocolate mixture to bowl with avocado. Whip for 1-2 minutes with electric mixer, until smooth consistency.

4) Stir in the cocoa powder and sugar. Whip 1 minute, until smooth.
5) Add the vanilla extract, cream, salt, and espresso. Whip again until smooth and fluffy, approximately 2 minutes.
6) Pour the batter over pie crust. Chill for 2 hours.
7) Serve with whipped cream!

Nutrition Values

- Calories: 265
- Fat: 4g
- Carbohydrates: 12g
- Protein: 1g
- Dietary Fiber: 1g

Cinnamon Apple Chips

(Prep time: 10 minutes\ Cook time: 120 minutes| 4 servings)

We don't really consider apples as anything but a healthy snack. Well, now, you can have your chips and eat 'em, too!

Ingredients:

- 2 organic apples
- Cinnamon

Preparation:

Preheat oven to 225F
1) Using a sharp knife or mandolin, slice the apples thinly.
2) Line cookie sheet with parchment paper. Arrange slices in single layer. Lightly sprinkle cinnamon over the slices.
3) Bake for an hour. Flip the slices over. Sprinkle a light layer of cinnamon over apple slices. Bake for another hour. (Apples should no longer moist by end of baking.)
4) Remove the chips. Cool for 10 minutes before eating.
5) Store in air tight container.

Nutrition Values

Calories: 175 Fat: 36g Carbohydrates: 16g Protein: 12g Dietary Fiber: 10g

Blueberry Smoothie

(Prep time: 10 minutes\ Cook time: 120 minutes| 10 ounce)

This blend is nothing short of Popeye's very own power-enhancing mixture!

Ingredients:

- ½ a frozen banana
- ¾ cup of frozen blueberries
- 1 handful of spinach leaves
- ¾ cup of nonfat honey Greek yogurt
- ⅔ cup of almond coconut milk
- 1 Tablespoon of hemp hearts
- 1 Tablespoon of vanilla whey protein powder
- 1 teaspoon of maca powder
- 1 teaspoon of maple syrup
- Bee pollen

Preparation:

1) Place all the ingredients in a blender. Pulse until smooth.
2) Chill 15 minutes to 2 hours. Enjoy!

Nutrition Values

Calories: 261 Fat: 4.2g Carbohydrates: 20g Protein: 10.1g Dietary Fiber: 4.6g

Candied Pecans

(Prep time: 10 minutes\ Cook time: 60 minutes| 2 serving)

This sweet treat is sure to turn the head of any lover of nuts!

Ingredients:

- 2 cups of pecans
- 1 egg white
- 1 Tablespoon of water

- ¼ cup of honey
- Pinch of sea salt
- Pinch of cinnamon

Preparation:

Preheat oven to 250F

1) Cover a cookie sheet with parchment paper.
2) In a medium bowl, blend the egg white and water until fluffy.
3) Add the honey, cinnamon, and salt. Stir. Add pecans to the bowl. Stir until evenly coated.
4) Using a slotted spoon, transfer pecans in single layer to cookie sheet.
5) Bake for 60 minutes. Stir every 15 minutes.
6) Spread nuts on glass surface to cool.

Nutrition Values

Calories: 190 Fat: 17g Carbohydrates: 10g Protein: 1g; Dietary Fiber: 5g

Blueberry Mug Muffin

(Prep time: 1 minute\ Cook time: 1 minute\ 1 serving)

A sweet treat for one!

Ingredients:

- 1 Tbsp cream cheese
- 1 large egg
- 2 Tbsp vanilla whey protein
- ¼ tsp baking powder
- $\frac{1}{8}$ tsp nutmeg
- ¼ cup fresh blueberries

Preparation:

1. Add the cream cheese to a large mug.
2. Heat in microwave 10 seconds. Stir until smooth.
3. Add the egg. Whisk with a fork to combine.
4. Add the whey powder, nutmeg, and baking powder to the mug. Mix well.
5. Add the blueberries. Stir.
6. Microwave 20 seconds. Cook at 15 second intervals if needed to cook longer.
7. Fork or spoon, can be used to enjoy this sweet treat.

Nutrition Values

- Calories: 242
- Fat: 15.1g
- Carbs: 6.3g
- Protein: 19.2g
- Dietary Fiber: 0.9g

Apple Tart

(Prep time: 30 minutes\ Cook time: 45 minutes\ 8 servings)

Apple tart is close to the heart. A classic for any diet routine.

Ingredients:

- 5 medium red apples
- ¼ cup sucralose based sweetener
- ¾ tsp cinnamon
- ⅛ tsp nutmeg
- 1 Tbsp unsalted butter
- 1 Cinnamon pie crust or pre-made pie shell

Preparation:

1. Cinnamon pie crust recipe is included in Breakfast section. Use that recipe or a pre-made pie shell.
2. Preheat oven to 350F.
3. Dice the apples into bite-size slices.
4. In a large bowl, combine the apple slices, sweetener, cinnamon, and nutmeg. Stir to coat the apple slices.
5. Spoon mixture into pie shell. Cut up the tablespoon of butter into small pieces. Place them on top of the apples.
6. Cover pie with top of pie crust.
7. Pierce top of pie in a few places to allow steam to escape.
8. Place on baking sheet. Bake 30 minutes.
9. Cover with aluminum foil and bake another 20 minutes, until apples are tender.
10. Cool the pie 30 minutes before slicing.

Nutrition Values

- Calories: 238
- Fat: 14.3g
- Carbs: 18.1g
- Protein: 8.2g
- Dietary Fiber: 3.1g

Berries With Chocolate Ganache

(Prep time: 10 minutes\ Cook time: 5 minutes\ 6 servings)

Waiting for a chocolate recipe? This recipe will fulfill all of your chocolaty dreams.

Ingredients:

- 1 cup strawberries
- 2 cups raspberries
- 2 cups blueberries
- ½ cup sugar-free chocolate chips
- ⅓ cup heavy cream
- ½ tsp pure vanilla extract

Preparation:

1. In a large bowl, combine the fruit. Stir.
2. Divide the fruit between 6 dessert bowls.
3. Boil a pot of water on medium heat. Place a glass bowl over the pot. Pour in the chocolate chips. Allow to melt. Stir in the cream. Remove from heat. Stir in the vanilla. Allow to cool slightly.
4. Pour over the fruit. Serve.

Nutrition Values

- Calories: 260
- Fat: 17.8g
- Carbs: 11.7g
- Protein: 2.3g
- Dietary Fiber: 7.4g

Caramelized Pear Custard

(Prep time: 10 minutes\ Cook time: 20 minutes\ 8 servings)

Caramelizing pears. Can you say drool?

Ingredients:

- 2 Tbsp butter
- 2 Tbsp Xylitol
- ¼ tsp ground cardamom
- 2 medium pears
- 3 eggs

- 2 egg yolks
- 2 cups heavy cream
- $\frac{1}{8}$ cup sugar-free low calorie maple syrup
- ½ tsp rum
- 1 tsp pure vanilla extract

Preparation:

Preheating oven to 375F

1. Peel the pears. Slice them in half.
2. In a sauce pan, over medium heat, melt the butter. Add the rum, xylitol and cardamom. Stir well.
3. Add the pears to sauce pan. Cover with sauce. Cook 4 minutes per side.
4. Transfer the pears and sauce to a deep glass dish.
5. In a small bowl, whisk the eggs, egg yolks, maple syrup, heavy cream, and vanilla until fully combined and smooth. Pour mixture over pears.
6. Bake 20 minutes, until golden brown and the custard has set.
7. Remove from oven. Cool slightly before serving.
8. Using a pastry brush, lightly brush the pears with maple syrup. Serve.

Nutrition Values

- Calories: 310
- Fat: 27g
- Carbs: 7.6g
- Protein: 4.4g
- Dietary Fiber: 1.3g

Chocolate Brownie Drops

(Prep time: 15 mins\ Cook time: 15 mins\ 12 servings)

These brownie drops are both healthy and sweet.

Ingredients:

- $\frac{1}{8}$ cup stone ground whole wheat pastry flour
- 2 Tbsp whole grain soy flour
- ¼ tsp baking powder
- ¼ cup unsweetened chocolate baking squares
- 6 Tbsp heavy cream
- 2 Tbsp unsalted butter
- 2 large eggs
- ¾ cup sucralose based sweetener

Preparation:

Preheat oven to 375F

1. Microwave the chocolate squares until almost melted. Add the butter. Stir until shinny. Set aside to cool.
2. Line a baking sheet with parchment paper.
3. In a large bowl, using an electric mixer, blend the butter until smooth. Add the sugar substitute. Blend again until smooth. Add the eggs, one at a time. Continue beating until smooth. Add the cooled chocolate to bowl. Continue beating.
4. In a separate bowl, whisk the flour, baking powder, and soy flour.
5. Pour in the flour mixture slowly. Beat until just combined.
6. Using a rounded spoon, spoon drops of batter onto the baking sheet.
7. Bake 5-6 minutes. Transfer to wire rack to cool. Serve.

Nutrition Values

- Calories: 104
- Fat: 9.4g
- Carbs: 3.9g
- Protein: 2.5g
- Dietary Fiber: 3.9g

Baked Pear Fans

(Prep time: 10 minutes\ Cook time: 40 minutes\ 4 servings)

While the recipe might seem bizarre, you will come to love the combination of these unique flavors.

Ingredients:

- 2 medium pears
- 1 Tbsp unsalted butter
- ¼ tsp black pepper
- ¼ tsp ginger
- ¼ tsp cinnamon
- 1 tsp tap water
- ¼ tsp pure vanilla extract

Preparation:

Preheat oven to 375F

1. You are going to make fans out of your pears. Make ¼ inch slices along the length of your half pear, starting ⅓ of an inch from the stem while cutting them all the way down to the bottom.
2. In a skillet, melt the butter. Add the lemon juice and water. Stir in the ginger, pepper, and cinnamon.
3. Place the pears in the skillet.
4. Cover with aluminum foil. Transfer skillet to oven. Bake 40 minutes. Turn the pears halfway through cooking.
5. Using a slotted spoon, transfer pears to serving plates.
6. Place skillet on stove. Stir in the vanilla. Simmer 1 minute.
7. Scoop the sauce over the pears. Serve.

Nutrition Values

- Calories: 80
- Fat: 3g
- Carbs: 11.5g
- Protein: 0.4g
- Dietary Fiber: 2.9g

Chocolate Frosty

(Prep time: 3 minutes\ Cook time: 0 minutes\ 1 serving)

A frosty! A chocolate one at that. Bring it on!

Ingredients:

- 2 Tbsp chocolate milk
- 2 Tbsp heavy cream
- 2 Tbsp sugar-free chocolate syrup
- ½ cup ice cubes

Preparation:

1. In a blender, combine the heavy cream, chocolate syrup, ice cubes. Blend until thick and smooth. Add a bit of chocolate milk for less thick consistency. Add more ice for a thicker consistency.
2. You could chill it for 20 minutes.

Nutrition Values

- Calories: 119
- Fat: 11.1g
- Carbs: 0.8g
- Protein: 1.6g
- Dietary Fiber: 1g

Ginger Flan

(Prep time: 180 minutes\ Cook time: 25 minutes\ 6 servings)

Unlike traditional pudding, this will give you a sweet taste and sensation of spice.

Ingredients:

- 3 egg yolks
- 2 egg
- 1½ cups heavy cream
- 1 cup tap water
- 8 packets sucralose based sweetener
- 1 tsp pure vanilla extract
- 3 tsp ground ginger

Preparation:

Preheat oven to 350F

1. Place a roasting pan on center shelf of oven. Fill to half with boiling water.
2. In a blender, combine the eggs, egg yolks, water, cream, sugar substitute, ginger, and vanilla. Blend until smooth.
3. Pass the sauce through a sieve. Pour into a 1-quart shallow baking dish.
4. Place the dish in the water bath in the oven. Bake 30-35 minutes.
5. Transfer to a cooling rack.
6. Once cooled, spray plastic wrap with non-stick cooking spray. Place it gently against the flan. Chill in the fridge 3 hours.
7. Once chilled, invert the baking dish and tap the flan onto a serving platter.

Nutrition Values

- Calories: 265
- Fat: 26g
- Carbs: 3.9g
- Protein: 4.6g
- Dietary Fiber: 0g

Coconut Cashew Bars

(Prep time: 10-15 minutes\ Cook time: 2 hours\ 8 servings)

A healthy nut bar you can make yourself. Satisfy a sweet tooth and healthy regime.

Ingredients:

- 1 cup almond flour
- 1 tsp cinnamon
- Pinch of salt
- ½ cup cashew nuts
- ¼ cup shredded coconut
- ¼ cup melted butter
- ¼ cup sugar-free maple syrup

Preparation:

1. In a large bowl, combine the flour, cinnamon, salt. Whisk briefly.
2. Smash the cashews. Add them with the coconut to the bowl.
3. Stir in the butter and maple syrup.
4. Line an 8x8 baking dish with parchment paper. Pour in the batter. Spread into an even layer.
5. Place in refrigerator. Chill 2 hours. Slice into bars.

Nutrition Values:

- Calories: 189.3
- Fat: 17.6g
- Carbs: 6.1g
- Protein: 4.4g
- Fiber: 2.1g
- Net Carbs: 4.0g

Choco Peanut Tart

(Prep time: 10-15 minutes\ Cook time: 30 minutes\ 4 servings)

Before the day ends, treat yourself with a tart.

Ingredients:

Crust

- ¼ cup flaxseed
- 2 Tbsp almond flour
- 1 Tbsp Erythritol
- 1 large egg (just need the egg white)

Middle Layer

- 4 Tbsp smooth peanut butter
- 2 Tbsp unsalted butter

Top Layer

- 1 medium avocado
- 4 Tbsp cocoa powder
- ¼ cup Erythritol
- ½ tsp pure vanilla extract
- ½ tsp cinnamon
- 2 Tbsp heavy cream

Preparation:

Preheat oven to 350F
1. Whisk the egg white.
2. In a large bowl, grind the flaxseed to a powdery consistency.
3. Add the almond flour, Erythritol. Stir in the egg white until crumbly.
4. Pour the mixture into a pie dish. Press in an even layer along bottom of pie dish. Bake for 8 minutes. Cool the crust completely before filling.
5. In a separate bowl, mash the avocado until smooth. Add the cocoa powder, Erythritol, cinnamon, vanilla extract, cream. Whisk until smooth.
6. In a separate bowl, melt the butter. Add peanut butter. Stir until smooth.
7. Pour the peanut butter batter in the pie dish. Spread in an even layer.
8. Pour the chocolate layer over the peanut butter layer. Smooth it out.
9. Refrigerator 1 hour.

Nutrition Values:

- Calories: 304.8
- Fat: 26.8g
- Carbs: 10.5g
- Protein: 9.8g
- Fiber: 6.6g
- Net Carbs: 3.9g

Brownies

(Prep time: 10 minutes\ Cook time: 20 minutes\ 8 large brownies)

Out of the hundreds of brownie recipes out there, this one is near perfect and delicious.

Ingredients:

- 1 Tbsp psyllium husk powder
- 2 cups almond flour
- 1 tsp baking powder
- ½ tsp salt
- ½ cup cocoa powder
- ⅓ cup Erythritol
- ¼ cup shredded coconut
- 2 large eggs
- ¼ cup maple syrup
- 2 Tbsp torani salted caramel

Preparation:

Preheat oven to 350F

1. Line an 8x8 baking pan with parchment paper. Grease with butter. Dust with cocoa powder.
2. In a large bowl, combine the husk powder, almond flour, baking powder, salt, cocoa powder, Erythritol, and shredded coconut. Whisk to combine.
3. In a separate bowl, whisk the eggs. Add the maple syrup, and salted caramel. Stir.
4. Fold the dry ingredients into the wet ingredients. Stir until just combined.
5. Bake 20 minutes.
6. Cool 30 minutes before slicing.

Nutrition:

- Calories: 258.1
- Fat: 23.7g
- Carbs: 10.4g
- Protein: 8.0g
- Fiber: 5.9g
- Net Carbs: 4.5g

Mini Vanilla Cloud Cupcakes

(Prep time: 10 minutes\ Cook time: 30-35 minutes\ 8 servings)

Guilt-free cupcakes.

Ingredients:

Cupcakes

- 6 large eggs, room temperature
- 6 Tbsp cream cheese, room temperature
- ½ tsp cream of tartar
- 2 tsp pure vanilla extract
- ¼ cup granulated stevia/Erythritol mixture

Frosting

- ½ cup cream cheese, room temperature
- 2 Tbsp butter, room temperature
- ⅓ cup granulated stevia/Erythritol mix
- 1 Tbsp pure vanilla extract

Preparation:

Preheat oven to 300F
1. Separate the eggs yolks and egg whites.
2. Spray 2 muffin tins with non-stick cooking spray.
3. In a bowl, using an electric mixer, beat the cream cheese until smooth. Add the egg yolks one at a time. Stir in sweetener and vanilla extract until smooth batter.
4. In a separate bowl, whip egg whites until fluffy. Stir in cream of tartar.
5. Combine the egg whites with the egg yolk batter. Fold in gently until combined.
6. Using an ice cream scoop, fill the muffin tin cups ¾ full.
7. Place tin in oven. Bake 30-35 minutes, until toothpick comes out dry.
8. Place on cooling rack. Cool completely before icing.

9. In a bowl, combine the cream cheese and butter. Whip with electric mixer until smooth. Add the sweetener and vanilla. Whip until smooth.
10. Ice the cupcakes. Serve.

Nutrition Values:

- Calories: 347.9
- Fat: 30.8g
- Carbs: 6.9g
- Protein: 9.25g
- Fiber: 3.5g
- Net Carbs: 3.38g

Pumpkin Pecan Pie Ice Cream

(Prep time: 10 minutes\ Cook time: 10-15 minutes\ 4 servings)

We all scream for ice cream.

Ingredients:

- ½ cup cottage cheese
- ½ cup pumpkin puree
- 2 cups coconut milk
- 3 large egg yolks
- ⅓ cup Erythritol
- ½ tsp Xanthan gum
- 20 drops liquid Stevia
- 1 tsp pure maple extract
- 1 tsp pumpkin spice
- ½ cup toasted pecans, chopped
- 2 Tbsp salted butter

Preparation:

1. In a skillet, melt some butter. Toast the pecans. Set aside to cool.
2. In a separate bowl, combine the cottage cheese, pumpkin puree, coconut milk, egg yolks. Blend with electric mixer.
3. Stir in toasted pecans, xanthan gum, pumpkin spice, liquid stevia, maple extract.
4. Pour the mixture into an ice cream machine.
5. Churn according to instruction of ice cream machine. Serve.

Nutrition Values:

- Calories: 248.3
- Fat: 22.3g
- Carbs: 7.1g
- Protein: 6.5g
- Fiber: 2.9g
- Net Carbs: 4.3g

Amaretti Cookies

(Prep time: 10 minutes\ Cook time: 16 minutes\ 16 Cookies)

Fruit-filled cookies are downright addictive.

Ingredients:

- 1 cup almond flour
- 2 Tbsp coconut flour
- ½ tsp baking powder
- ¼ tsp cinnamon
- ½ tsp salt
- ½ cup Erythritol
- 1 Tbsp shredded coconut
- 4 Tbsp coconut oil
- 2 large eggs
- ½ tsp pure vanilla extract
- ½ tsp almond extract
- 2 Tbsp sugar-free jam

Preparation:

Preheat oven to 350F

1. Line a cookie sheet with parchment paper.
2. In a bowl, combine the almond flour, coconut flour, baking powder, cinnamon, salt, Erythritol. Whisk together.
3. In another bowl, add the coconut oil. Stir to soften it. Stir in one egg at a time. Add the vanilla. Stir until combined.
4. Add dry ingredients to wet ingredients. Stir until just combined.
5. Using a tablespoon, scoop cookie dough onto cookie sheet; 1 inch apart.
6. Dab your finger in water, and press an indent in the middle of the dough.
7. Bake 16 minutes.
8. Place on a cooling rack. Cool 30 minutes.
9. Add 1 teaspoon of jam to indent in cookie. Garnish with shredded coconut.

Nu

trition Values:

- Calories: 85.7
- Fat: 7.9g
- Carbs: 2.5g
- Protein: 2.4g
- Fiber: 1.3g
- Net Carbs: 1.2g

Chocolate Dipped Macaroons

(Prep time: 10 minutes\ Cook time: 15 minutes\ 12 Macaroons)

Macaroons are really awesome for their gooey consistency and heart-melting flavor.

Ingredients:

- 1 cup shredded coconut
- 1 large egg white
- ¼ cup Erythritol
- ½ tsp almond extract
- Pinch of salt
- ½ cup sugar-free chocolate
- 2 Tbsp coconut oil

Preparation:

Preheat oven to 350F

1. Line a cookie sheet with parchment paper. Sprinkle the shredded coconut in a thin layer over the cookie sheet.
2. Bake 5 minutes. Watch the oven. Remove when golden brown.
3. Once the coconut is toasted, set aside. In a bowl, beat the eggs with an electric mixer until fluffy. Mix in the Erythritol and salt.
4. Add the cooled down toasted coconut to the batter. Stir well.
5. Drop 1 tablespoon of batter onto cookie sheet, 1 inch apart.
6. Bake 15 minutes, turn pan around. Bake another 15 minutes.
7. Remove from oven. Cool on pan 5 minutes, transfer to cooling rack to cool completely. Melt the chocolate.
8. Once cooled, dip macaroons in melted chocolate. Let them set 5 minutes.

Nutrition Values:

- Calories: 73.2
- Fat: 7.3g
- Carbs: 2.7g
- Protein: 1.0g
- Fiber: 1.7g
- Net Carbs: 1.0g

Chapter 6: Fulfilling Snacks

Balsamic Rosemary Roasted Vegetables

(Prep time: 10 minutes\ Cook time: 60 minutes| 4 servings)

Whip up these rosemary coated vegetables for a kick to your immunity.

Ingredients:

- 2 cups of butternut squash, chopped in small cubes
- 1½ cups of broccoli florets
- ½ red onion, chopped in bite-size pieces
- 1 zucchini, chopped in bite-size pieces
- ½ red bell pepper, chopped in bite-size pieces
- 1 garlic clove, minced
- 2 Tablespoons of olive oil
- 1 Tablespoon of balsamic vinegar
- 1½ Tablespoons of fresh rosemary
- ½ Tablespoon of sea salt
- ½ teaspoon of black pepper

Preparation:

Preheat oven to 425F
4) Line a cookie sheet with parchment paper.
5) In a large bowl, whisk the vinegar, oil, salt and pepper.
6) Toss the vegetables in the oil until evenly coated.
7) Spread the mixture in a single layer on cookie sheet.
8) Bake for 45 - 60 minutes, until fork tender. Serve hot.

Nutrition Values

- Calories: 98
- Fat: 2.1g
- Carbohydrates: 19g
- Protein: 3g
- Dietary Fiber: 5g

Spiced and Crispy Carrot Chips

(Prep time: 50 minutes\ Cook time: 10 minutes| 1-2 servings)

Yes, you read that right. These paprika and cumin covered carrot chips might sound weird at first, but they are blast to have.

Ingredients:

- 3 cups of carrots sliced paper thin
- 2 Tablespoons of olive oil
- 2 teaspoons of ground cumin
- ½ teaspoon of smoked paprika
- Pinch of salt

Preparation:

Preheat oven to 400F

1) Cover a cookie sheet with parchment paper.
2) Using a sharp knife or mandolin, slice carrots paper thin.
3) In a large bowl, combine carrot slices with oil, cumin, paprika, and salt. Stir to evenly coat.
4) Place the pieces in a single layer on the cookie sheet.
5) Bake 8 - 10 minutes, until crispy.

Nutrition Values

Calories: 280 Fat: 0g Carbohydrates: 0g Protein: 0g Dietary Fiber: 0g

Eggplant Caponata

(Prep time: 10 minutes\ Cook time: 20 minutes| 2 servings)

Another surprising recipe using an Eggplant, that leaves you fulfilled.

Ingredients:

- 2 Tablespoons of olive oil
- 3 garlic cloves, minced
- 2 onions, finely diced
- 4 cups of chopped eggplant
- 4 cups of chopped tomatoes
- 3 Tablespoons of white vinegar
- 2 Tablespoons of capers
- ½ cup of chopped up basil

Preparation:

1) In a large frying pan, drizzle oil over bottom of pan. Sauté the onions and garlic, until soft and translucent.
2) Cut up the eggplant. Add to the frying pan. Season with salt.
3) Cook eggplant 5 minutes, until fork tender. Drizzle oil over eggplant.
4) Add the tomatoes.
5) Stir in the vinegar.
6) Simmer 10 minutes, until the tomatoes are tender.
7) Serve in bowls. Garnish with basil and capers.

Nutrition Values

Calories: 175
Fat: 0g
Carbohydrates: 3g
Protein: 10g
Dietary Fiber: 5g

Sautéed Mushrooms

(Prep time: 10 minutes\ Cook time: 20 minutes| 2 servings)

Mushrooms...what can I say about Mushrooms? These are our favorite little fungi we love to eat! Yes, even as a snack.

Ingredients:

- 2 Tablespoons of butter
- 1 Tablespoon of olive oil
- 1½ pound of gourmet mushrooms
- 4 garlic cloves, diced
- ⅓ cup of white wine
- Pinch of salt

Preparation:

1) In a large, heavy skillet, heat up the oil and half the butter.
2) When the pan is almost smoking, add the mushrooms.
3) Stir the mushroom until soft and fork tender.
4) Add rest of the butter.
5) Stir in the garlic.
6) Add the white wine.
7) Once liquid has been absorbed, season with salt. Serve hot.

Nutrition Values

Calories: 124
Fat: 2g
Carbohydrates: 17g
Protein: 12g
Dietary Fiber: 0g

Sautéed Radishes

You may be pleasantly surprised by experiencing this unique blend of multiple flavors from radishes.

Ingredients:

- 2 bunches of radishes, about 20 in total
- 1 Tablespoon of olive oil
- 1 teaspoon of butter
- 2 Tablespoons of honey
- 2 Tablespoons of white balsamic
- ¼ teaspoon of sea salt

Preparation:

Preheat oven to 350F
1) Slice the radishes to ¼ inch thickness.
2) In a large frying pan, heat the olive oil. Sauté the radishes.
3) Pour them into a baking dish.
4) In the same frying pan, melt the butter.
5) Add the honey. Stir in the balsamic vinegar and pinch of salt.
6) Pour the glaze over the radishes. Stir until evenly coated.
7) Heat the radishes in the oven for 15 minutes. Serve hot.

Nutrition Values

Calories: 25
Fat: 0.4g
Carbohydrates: 5g
Protein: 1g
Dietary Fiber: 2.4g

Roasted Heirloom Carrots

(Prep time: 10 minutes\ Cook time: 45 minutes| 3-4 servings)

These Roasted Heirloom carrots are crafted with the care they deserve for the taste buds that deserve them!

Ingredients:

- 1 bunch of fine heirloom carrots
- 1 Tablespoon of fresh thyme leaves
- ½ Tablespoon of coconut oil
- 1 Tablespoon of maple syrup
- $\frac{1}{8}$ cup of freshly squeezed orange juices
- $\frac{1}{8}$ teaspoon of sea salt

Preparation:

Preheat oven to 350F
1) Line a cookie sheet with parchment paper.
2) Thoroughly wash the carrots, remove any green parts.
3) In a small bowl, combine the coconut oil, maple syrup, orange juice, and sea salt. Stir until combined.
4) Pour mixture over carrots.
5) Spread the carrots out in a thin layer on the cookie sheet.
6) Sprinkle the carrots with thyme.
7) Roast for 45 minutes, or until fork tender.
8) Garnish with fresh thyme. Serve warm.

Nutrition Values

Calories: 70

Fat: 3g

Carbohydrates: 11g

Protein: 1g

Dietary Fiber: 3g

<u>Beans With Crushed Almonds</u>

(Prep time: 10 minutes\ Cook time: 20 minutes| 4 servings)

Get the health benefits of green beans in the form of a snack that is designed for a Paleo buff!

Ingredients:

- 1 pound of fresh green beans, ends trimmed
- 1½ Tablespoons of olive oil
- ¼ teaspoon of salt
- 1½ Tablespoons of fresh dill, minced
- Juice from 1 lemon
- ¼ cup of crushed almonds
- Sea salt for garnish

Preparation:

Preheat oven to 400F
1) Line a cookie sheet with parchment paper.
2) Toss green beans with olive oil. Season with salt.
3) Spread the green beans in a single layer across the cookie sheet.
4) Roast 10 minutes. Stir once.
5) Continue cooking for 8 – 10 minutes, until fork tender.
6) Remove from oven.
7) Place in a bowl. Drizzle lemon juice over the beans. Stir.
8) Garnish with fresh dill, crushed almonds, and sea salt.

Nutrition Values

Calories: 120

Carbohydrates: 13g

Dietary Fiber: 5g

Fat: 8g

Protein: 4g

Cauliflower Couscous with Apricots and Cashews

(Prep time: 20 minutes\ Cook time: 20 minutes| 4-6 servings)

Don't judge it before you taste it, as it just might turn out to be one of your favorite dishes.

Ingredients:

- 2 heads of cauliflower, diced in florets
- ½ cup of roasted cashew nut
- ⅓ cup of apricots, cut into raisin-size pieces
- 4 scallions, finely chopped

- 4 Tablespoons of fresh parsley, chopped
- 2 Tablespoons of fresh cilantro, chopped
- ¼ teaspoon of red pepper flakes
- Pinch of salt and pepper

For the Dressing

- 2 Tablespoons of dates, mashed
- 2 Tablespoons of olive oil
- 2 Tablespoons of water

- 1 Tablespoon of fresh lemon juice
- 2 Tablespoons of fresh orange juice
- 2 teaspoons of fresh ginger, grated
- ½ teaspoon of ground cinnamon
- Pinch of salt and pepper

Preparation:

Preheat oven to 425F

1) Drizzle oil lightly over large baking sheet.
2) Place the cauliflower florets in a food processor. Pulse until a rice-like consistency is achieved.
3) Spread out the cauliflower in a thin layer on the baking sheet.
4) Bake for 15-20 minutes, stirring every 5 minutes.
5) Remove from oven. Allow to cool completely.
6) Mash the dates using a food processor.

7) Dressing: In a large bowl, combine the mashed dates, olive oil, water, lemon juice, orange juice, ginger, cinnamon, salt, and pepper. Whisk to combine.

8) Pour in the cooled cauliflower. Stir until evenly coated with dressing.

9) Serve.

Nutrition Values

- Calories: 570
- Fat: 21g
- Carbohydrates: 25g
- Protein: 17g
- Dietary Fiber: 6.3g

Apricot-Apple Cloud

(Prep time: 65 minutes\ Cook time: 10 minutes\ 6 servings)

Even though the apricot apple cloud seems geared towards children, don't let it fool you. It is a snack worthy of any Atkins follower.

Ingredients:

- 1½ cups heavy cream
- 2 cups unsweetened applesauce baby food
- 2 Tbsp sucralose based sweetener

Preparation:

1. In a large bowl, using an electric mixer, whip the heavy cream. Add the sugar substitute. Beat until firm peaks form.
2. Gently fold in applesauce. Stir until combined.
3. Pour into 6 individual serving bowls.
4. Chill for 1 hour. Serve.

Nutrition Values

- Calories: 9.9
- Fat: 22.4
- Carbs: 25g
- Protein: 1.5g
- Dietary Fiber: 1.1g

Artichoke With Three Cheeses

(Prep time: 20 minutes\ Cook time: 40 minutes\ 4 servings)

Yet another intelligent way to get you to eat your green vegetable. Try not to gobble it.

Ingredients:

- 2 cups artichoke hearts
- ½ cup vegetable broth
- 3 Tbsp extra virgin olive oil
- 1 tsp lemon juice
- 2 garlic cloves, minced
- Fresh parsley, chopped
- Fresh basil, chopped
- ½ cup shredded Fontina cheese
- ½ cup of shredded Swiss cheese
- ½ cup shredded Parmesan cheese

Preparation:

Preheat oven to 400F

1. Arrange artichokes in single layer of a deep baking dish.
2. Drizzle oil, lemon juice, garlic, vegetable broth over the artichokes.
3. Start with fontina cheese, then Swiss cheese, parmesan cheese last.
4. Cover baking dish with aluminum foil. Bake 15 minutes.
5. Remove foil. Bake an additional 15 minutes, until cheese is golden and bubbly.
6. Remove from oven. Let it cool to room temperature. Serve.

Nutrition Values

- Calories: 57
- Fat: 14g
- Carbs: 3g
- Protein: 4g
- Dietary Fiber: 2.6g

Peanut Butter Granola Bar with Strawberries And Yogurt Parfait

(Prep time: 5 minutes\ Cook time: 0 minutes\ 1 serving)

Granola bars are an excellent source of energy and combined with yogurt and strawberries, they can turn into a great Atkins suitable snack.

Ingredients:

- 1 cup plain Greek yogurt
- 1 Atkins Peanut Butter Granola Bar
- 5 strawberries, sliced

Preparation:

1. Place the granola bar in a baggie. Break up into small pieces.
2. Spoon a layer of yogurt in bottom of a dish.
3. Add a layer of smashed granola bar.
4. Spoon in a layer of yogurt.
5. Top with strawberries.
6. Serve immediately or chill in refrigerator.

Nutrition Values

- Calories: 314
- Fat: 9.5g
- Carbs: 12.6g
- Protein: 24.1g
- Dietary Fiber: 6.8g

Blackberry Peach Compote

(Prep time: 10 minutes\ Cook time: 20 minutes\ 12 servings)

This can be considered as both a snack and a desert.

Ingredients:

- ¼ cup Sauvignon Blanc wine
- 2 Tbsp Xylitol
- 1 tsp ground ginger
- 1 tsp Cinnamon
- 3 medium peaches
- ¼ cup blackberries
- ½ tsp thick it up

Preparation:

1. In a large saucepan, combine the wine, Xylitol, ginger, peaches, and cinnamon.
2. Simmer for 15 minutes.
3. Add the blackberries. Simmer another 5 minutes, until berries are tender.
4. Stir in the thick it up. Simmer approximately 5 minutes.
5. Remove from heat. Cool to room temperature. Serve.

Nutrition Values

- Calories: 35
- Fat: 0.2g
- Carbs: 4.2g
- Protein: 0.5g
- Dietary Fiber: 3.4g

Baked Brie

(Prep time: 5 minutes\ Cook time: 10 minutes\ 6 servings)

Melted cheese. Who could resist?

Ingredients:

- 8 oz Brie wheel cheese
- ¼ cup pine nuts

Preparation:

Heat oven to 450F

1. Trip top of white rind off cheese.
2. Cover top with pine nuts.
3. Place cheese on aluminum foil pan or pie dish.
4. Bake 10 minutes. Serve.

Nutrition Values

- Calories: 144
- Fat: 12.1g
- Carbs: 2.g
- Protein: 8.2g
- Dietary Fiber: 0.1g

Indian Chicken Curry

(Prep time: 8 minutes\ Cook time: 20 minutes\ 6 servings)

This curry is designed to give you the flavor of core Indian curries.

Ingredients:

- 3 Tbsp unsalted butter
- 2 garlic cloves, minced
- 4 chicken breasts, boneless, skinless
- 1 tsp cumin
- ½ tsp coriander
- ½ tsp ground ginger
- ¼ tsp crushed red pepper flakes
- ½ cup chicken broth
- ⅓ cup heavy cream
- Fresh cilantro

Preparation:

1. In a large skillet, melt the butter. Sauté the garlic for 2 minutes.
2. Add the chicken breasts. Cook thoroughly.
3. Once cooked, remove the chicken and cut into chunks. Return to the pan.
4. Pour in the chicken broth, cumin, coriander, ginger, red pepper flakes.
5. Turn down the heat to medium-low. Simmer 5 minutes.
6. Stir in the cream. Simmer another 3 minutes.
7. Serve in bowls over rice. Garnish with fresh cilantro.

Nutrition Values

- Calories: 413
- Fat: 22.1g
- Carbs: 1g
- Protein: 49.1g
- Dietary Fiber: 0.3g

Avocado Salsa

(Prep time: 10 minutes\ Cook time: 0 minutes\ 4 servings)

Avocados are really great, turning it into a salsa, even greater.

Ingredients:

- 1 red tomato
- ⅛ cup fresh cilantro, rough chopped
- 1 red onion, diced
- ½ jalapeno pepper, diced
- 2 avocadoes, diced
- 2-3 Tbsp fresh lime juice
- Pinch of salt and fresh ground black pepper

Preparation:

1. Chop all the vegetables.
2. Add them to a bowl.
3. Squeeze in the lime juice. Season with salt and pepper. Stir.
4. Refrigerate for 30 minutes. Serve.

Nutrition Values

- Calories: 71
- Fat: 5.3g
- Carbs: 3.3g
- Protein: 1.1g
- Dietary Fiber: 3g

Chicken Wings

(Prep time: 10 minutes\ Cook time: 35 minutes\ 8 servings)

A delicious treat.

Ingredients:

- ½ serving all purpose low carb baking mix
- 2 Tbsp chili powder
- 1 tsp cayenne pepper
- 2 tsp yellow mustard seed
- 2 tsp salt
- 12-16 chicken wings

Preparation:

Preheat oven to 450F

1. Rinse the chicken wings.
2. Line a baking sheet with aluminum foil. Spray with non-stick cooking spray.
3. Take a Ziploc bag, add the baking mix, chili powder, cayenne pepper, mustard seed, salt. Place the wings in the bag. Massage the chicken wings through the bag to coat them with seasoning.
4. Transfer to baking sheet. Cook 30-35 minutes, until golden brown.
5. Serve immediately.

Nutrition Values

- Calories: 276
- Fat: 18.5g
- Carbs: 3.4g
- Protein: 22.4g
- Dietary Fiber: 0.3g

Cauliflower Mushroom Risotto

(Prep time: 10 minutes\ Cook time: 10 minutes\ 2 servings)

A unique Italian dish with the warm flavors of mushroom and cauliflower, and healthy.

Ingredients:

- 1 Tbsp olive oil
- 2 garlic cloves, minced
- 4 baby bella mushrooms, diced
- 1 cup chicken broth
- 2 cups riced cauliflower
- ¼ cup parmesan cheese
- ¼ cup heavy cream
- 1 tsp tarragon
- Pinch of salt and pepper

Preparation:

1. In a blender, process the cauliflower until rice-like consistency.
2. In a skillet, heat the olive oil. Sauté the garlic, mushrooms for 3 minutes.
3. Pour in the chicken broth and cauliflower. Stir well. Simmer 5 minutes.
4. Once the liquid has cooked away, add the parmesan cheese and tarragon, salt, and pepper. Stir well. Stir in the cream. Keep stirring until the cheese has melted.
5. Serve hot.

Nutrition Values:

- Calories: 245.5
- Fat: 20g
- Carbs: 8.5g
- Protein: 7g
- Fiber: 2.5g
- Net Carbs: 6g

Coconut Orange Creamsicle Fat Bombs

(Prep time: 2-3 hours\ Cook time: nil\ 10 Fat bombs)

Enjoy a savory combination of coconut and orange in this fat bomb recipe.

Ingredients:

- ½ cup coconut oil
- ½ cup heavy whipping cream
- ¼ cup cream cheese
- 1 tsp orange vanilla Mio
- 10 drops liquid Stevia

Preparation:

1. Add the coconut oil to a blender. Pulse until smooth.
2. Add the whip cream. Pulse until combined.
3. Add the cream cheese. Pulse until smooth.
4. Add the orange Milo and Stevia. Pulse until smooth.
5. Spoon the mixture into silicon tray mold or ice cube tray. Freeze 3 hours.
6. Pop out to eat. Store uneaten bombs in a bag in the freezer.

Nutrition Values:

- Calories: 176
- Fat: 20g
- Carbs: 0.7g
- Protein: 0.8g
- Fiber: 0g
- Net Carbs: 0.7g

Corndog Muffins

(Prep time: 10 minutes \ Cook time: 15 minutes\ 20 Muffins)

Turn your ordinary muffin into a delightful meaty combination with these cute muffins.

Ingredients:

- ½ cup blanched almond flour
- ½ cup flaxseed meal
- 1 Tbsp psyllium husk powder
- 3 Tbsp swerve sweetener
- ¼ tsp salt
- ¼ tsp baking powder
- ¼ cup melted butter
- 1 egg
- ¼ cup coconut milk
- ⅓ cup sour cream
- 3 all beef hot dogs

Preparation:

Preheat oven to 375F
1. In a bowl, add the almond flour, flaxseed, husk powder, granulated sweetener, salt, and baking powder. Whisk together.
2. In a separate bowl, combine the egg, coconut milk. Whisk together. Add the butter. Stir until combined. Add the sour cream. Stir until combined.
3. Add the dry ingredients to the wet ingredients. Stir until a smooth batter forms.
4. Grease a 12 mini muffin tin.
5. Slice the hot dogs into 4 sections.
6. Fill the muffin cup half way. Add the sliced hot dog to the batter.
7. Bake 12 minutes.
8. Then broil 1-2 minutes, until golden brown. Serve.

Nutrition Values:

- Calories: 78.5
- Fat: 6.8g
- Carbs: 2.1g
- Protein: 2.4g
- Fiber: 1.5g
- Net Carbs: 0.7g

Layered Fried Queso Blanco

(Prep time: 10 minutes \ Cook time: 10 minutes\ multiple Servings)

Think frying up your cheese might be a bad idea? Think again.

Ingredients:

- ½ cup Queso Blanco
- 1½ Tbsp olive oil
- Pinch red pepper flakes or salt and pepper

Preparation:

1. Cut the cheese into cubes. Chill in the freezer as you heat the oil.
2. In a skillet, heat the olive oil. Once the pan is hot, add the cubes of cheese.
3. As it cooks it will melt. Once it is golden brown on one side, flip it over. Press down against the cheese to flatten it slightly and push out the oil. Once it is golden brown on both sides, tilt the edges against the pan and cook those until golden brown. It will seal the cheese into a square.
4. Remove from pan. Place on paper towel. Pat lightly. Slice into cubes again.
5. Sprinkle red pepper flakes or salt and pepper over the cubes. Serve immediately.

Nutrition Values:

- Calories: 525
- Fat: 43g
- Carbs: 4g
- Protein: 30g
- Fiber: 2g
- Net Carbs: 2g

Raspberry Lemon Popsicles

(Prep time: 10-15 minutes\ Cook time: 2 hours\ 6 servings)

How about a refreshing ice cream now?

Ingredients:

- 1 cup of raspberries
- Juice from ½ a lemon
- ¼ cup coconut oil
- 1 cup coconut milk
- ¼ cup sour cream
- ¼ cup heavy cream
- ½ tsp Guar Gum
- 20 drops liquid Stevia

Preparation:

1. Combine all the ingredients in a blender. Pulse until smooth. Strain the liquid.
2. Pour mixture into popsicle molds. Freeze 2 hours.
3. If stuck, run the mold under hot water briefly.

Nutrition Values:

- Calories: 150.5
- Fat: 16.0g
- Carbs: 3.3g
- Protein: 0.5
- Fiber: 1.3g
- Net Carbs: 2.0g

Neapolitan Fat Bombs

(Prep time: 15-30 minutes\ Cook time: 1 hour\ 24 servings)

Try out this recipe to satisfy a sweet craving.

Ingredients:

- ½ cup butter
- ½ cup coconut oil
- ½ cup sour cream
- ½ cup cream cheese
- 2 Tbsp liquid stevia
- 2 Tbsp cocoa powder
- 1 tsp pure vanilla extract
- 2 strawberries

Preparation:

1. In a blender, add the butter, coconut oil, sour cream, cream cheese. Pulse until smooth.
2. Set out 3 bowls. Add cocoa powder to a bowl. Add vanilla extract to another bowl. Add strawberries to a bowl. Mash them.
3. Pour the mixture evenly between the 3 bowls. Stir each mixture until smooth.
4. Pour vanilla mixture into bottom of silicon mold or ice cube tray. Freeze for 30 minutes. Place other bowls in the fridge. Pour the chocolate layer in the silicon mold or ice cube tray. Freeze 30 minutes. Pour the strawberry layer into the silicon mold or ice cube tray. Freeze 2 hours. Ready to serve.

Nutrition Values:

- Calories: 102.2
- Fat: 10.9g
- Carbs: 0.6g
- Protein: 0.6g
- Fiber: 0.2g
- Net Carbs: 0.4g

No Bake Chocolate Peanut Butter Balls

(Prep time: 20 minutes \ Cook time: nil\ 8 Fat bombs)

Don't even try to resist this treat.

Ingredients:

- ¼ cup cocoa powder
- 4 Tbsp Peanut Butter Fit Powder
- 5 Tbsp shelled hemp seeds
- 2 Tbsp heavy cream
- ½ cup coconut oil
- 1 tsp pure vanilla extract
- 28 drops liquid stevia
- ¼ cup unsweetened shredded coconut

Preparation:

1. In a bowl, crush the hemp seeds. Add the cocoa powder, fit powder. Stir. Add the coconut oil. Stir together until a paste forms.
2. Stir in the heavy cream, liquid stevia, and vanilla. Keep mixing until it forms a dough consistency.
3. Pinch off dough to make 1 inch round balls. Roll in unsweetened shredded coconut. Chill 30 minutes. Serve.

Nutrition Values:

- Calories: 208.3
- Fat: 20.0g
- Carbs: 3.1g
- Protein: 4.4g
- Fiber: 2.4g
- Net Carbs: 0.8g

Pizza Fat Bombs

(Prep time: 10 minutes\ Cook time: nil\ 6 Fat Bombs)

Why not fulfill your macronutrient needs by savoring pizza flavored fat bombs.

Ingredients:

- ¼ cup cream cheese
- 12 slices of pepperoni
- 6 pitted black olives
- 2 Tbsp sun dried tomato pesto
- 2 Tbsp fresh basil, chopped
- Pinch of salt and pepper

Preparation:

1. Dice up the pepperoni. Dice the black olives.
2. In a bowl, combine the cream cheese and tomato pesto. Stir in the pepperoni, black olives, and basil. Mash it all with a fork.
3. Pinch off some mixture, roll into 1 inch balls.
4. Place on a tray. Freeze 20 minutes. Serve.

Nutrition Values:

- Calories: 110.0
- Fat: 10.5g
- Carbs: 1.5g
- Protein: 2.3g
- Fiber: 0.2g
- Net Carbs: 1.3g

Sage and Cheddar Waffles

(Prep time: 10 minutes \ Cook time: 10 minutes\ 12 servings)

This delicious recipe is full of nutrition and you will like it.

Ingredients:

- ⅓ cup sifted coconut flour
- 3 tsp baking powder
- 1 tsp dried ground sage
- ½ tsp salt
- ¼ tsp garlic powder
- 2 eggs
- 2 cups canned coconut milk
- ¼ cup water
- 3 Tbsp melted coconut oil
- 1 cup shredded cheddar cheese

Preparation:

Preheat waffle iron.

1. In a bowl, combine the coconut flour, baking powder, sage, salt, garlic powder, and shredded cheese. Whisk together.
2. In a separate bowl, whisk the eggs. Add the coconut milk, water, melted coconut oil. Whisk briskly to combine. Add the dry ingredients to the wet. Stir until a batter forms.
3. Pour ⅓ scoop of batter onto waffle iron.
4. Close the iron. Cook until steam rises, 5-6 minutes.
5. Serve.

Nutrition Values:

- Calories: 213.97
- Fat: 17.21g
- Carbs: 9.2g
- Protein: 6.52g
- Fiber: 5.4g
- Net Carbs: 3.81g

Chapter 7: Paleo Diet Epic Meal Plan

Meal Plans

Please note that the recipes found in the following Meal Plans might not be found in the provided recipes in this book. The meal plan is provided as a rough guide on how to approach your diet. If you wish, you can alter any of the dishes from the 40 recipes provided in the book to create your own favorite diet routine!

Week 1: Shopping List and Meal Plan

- Bananas, Eggs, Almond Butter, Coconut Flour, Cinnamon
- Baking Powder, Pure vanilla extract, Salt, Dark Chocolate
- Extra Virgin Coconut Oil, Raw Honey, Large Eggs
- Coconut Milk, Pure vanilla extract, Coconut Milk, Spinach
- Tartar Cream, Baking Soda, Sea Salt, Carrots
- Bell Pepper, Onion, Garlic, Cumin Seeds, Paprika
- Avocado, Lime, Salsa, Roma Tomatoes, Cucumber, Cilantro
- Nitrate Free Bacon, Butternut Squash, Sage, Pepper
- Turkey, Sweet Potatoes, Eggplant, Chili Powder
- Oregano, Cardamom, Tarragon Flakes, Almond Milk, Rosemary

Day 1(Totals: Calories: 1238; Fat: 63g; Carbs: 37.8g; Protein: 48G)

Breakfast:

Chocolate Chunk Banana Bread

(Calories: 250; Fat: 18.2g; Carbs: 19.4g; Protein: 6.8g)

Snack

Crispy Balsamic Rosemary Roasted Vegetables

(Calories: 98; Fat: 2.18g; Carbs: 19g; Protein: 3g)

Lunch

Taco Salad In Mason Jar

(Calories: 177; Fat: 9.14g; Carbs: 9.8g; Protein: 16g)

Snack

Crispy Carrot Chips

(Calories: 280; Fat: 0g; Carbs: 0g; Protein: 0g)

Dinner

Skillet Chicken Thighs With Butternut Squash

(Calories: 323; Fat: 19g; Carbs: 15g; Protein: 12g)

Dessert

Graham Crackers

(Calories: 110; Fat: 0g; Carbs: 10; Protein: 0g)

Day 2(Totals: Calories: 886; Fat: 72g; Carbs: 78g; Protein: 36.9g)

Breakfast:

Coconut Flour Pancakes

(Calories: 65; Fat: 4.2g; Carbs: 3.6g; Protein: 2.5g)

Snack

Eggplant Caponata

(Calories: 98; Fat: 2.18g; Carbs: 19g; Protein: 3g)

Lunch

Crunchy Lettuce Tacos With Chipotle Chicken

(Calories: 175; Fat: 0g; Carbs: 3; Protein: 10g)

Snack

Sautéed Mushrooms

(Calories: 124; Fat: 2g; Carbs: 17g; Protein: 12g)

Dinner

Turkey Potato Casserole W/Eggplant and Tomato

(Calories: 278; Fat: 2.6g; Carbs: 15g; Protein: 28g)

Dessert

Mango Chia Seed Pudding

(Calories: 146; Fat: 26g; Carbs: 15g; Protein: 23g)

Day 3(Totals: Calories: 1238; Fat: 63g; Carbs: 37.8g; Protein: 48g)

Breakfast:

Chocolate Chunk Banana Bread

(Calories: 250; Fat: 18.2g; Carbs: 19.4g; Protein: 6.8g)

Snack

Crispy Balsamic Rosemary Roasted Vegetables

(Calories: 98; Fat: 2.18g; Carbs: 19g; Protein: 3g)

Lunch

Taco Salad In Mason Jar

(Calories: 177; Fat: 9.14g; Carbs: 9.8g; Protein: 16g)

Snack

Crispy Carrot Chips

(Calories: 280; Fat: 0g; Carbs: 0g; Protein: 0g)

Dinner

Skillet Chicken Thighs With Butternut Squash

(Calories: 323; Fat: 19g; Carbs: 15g; Protein: 12g)

Dessert

Graham Crackers

(Calories: 110; Fat: 0g; Carbs: 10; Protein: 0g)

Day 4(Totals: 886 Calories; Fat: 72g; Carbs: 78g; Protein: 36.9g)

Breakfast:

Coconut Flour Pancakes

(Calories: 65; Fat: 4.2g; Carbs: 3.6g; Protein: 2.5g)

Snack

Eggplant Caponata

(Calories: 98; Fat: 2.18g; Carbs: 19g; Protein: 3g)

Lunch

Lettuce Tacos With Chipotle Chicken

(Calories: 175; Fat: 0g; Carbs: 3; Protein: 10g)

Snack

Sautéed Mushrooms

(Calories: 124; Fat: 2g; Carbs: 17g; Protein: 12g)

Dinner

Turkey Potato Casserole W/Eggplant and Tomato

(Calories: 278; Fat: 2.6g; Carbs: 15g; Protein: 28g)

Dessert

Mango Chia Seed Pudding

(Calories: 146; Fat: 26g; Carbs: 15g; Protein: 23g)

Day 5(Totals: Calories: 1238; Fat: 63g; Carbs: 37.8g; Protein: 48g)

Breakfast:

Chocolate Chunk Banana Bread

(Calories: 250; Fat: 18.2g; Carbs: 19.4g; Protein: 6.8g)

Snack

Balsamic Rosemary Roasted Vegetables

(Calories: 98; Fat: 2.18g; Carbs: 19g; Protein: 3g)

Lunch

Taco Salad In Mason Jar

(Calories: 177; Fat: 9.14g; Carbs: 9.8g; Protein: 16g)

Snack

Crispy Carrot Chips

(Calories: 280; Fat: 0g; Carbs: 0g; Protein: 0g)

Dinner

Skillet Chicken Thighs With Butternut Squash

(Calories: 323; Fat: 19g; Carbs: 15g; Protein: 12g)

Dessert

Graham Crackers

(Calories: 110; Fat: 0g; Carbs: 10; Protein: 0g)

Day 6(Totals: 886; Fat: 72g; Carbs: 78g protein: 36.9)

Breakfast:

Coconut Flour Pancakes

(Calories: 65; Fat: 4.2g; Carbs: 3.6g; Protein: 2.5g)

Snack

Eggplant Caponata

(Calories: 98; Fat: 2.18g; Carbs: 19g; Protein: 3g)

Lunch

Lettuce Tacos With Chipotle Chicken

(Calories: 175; Fat: 0g; Carbs: 3; Protein: 10g)

Snack

Sautéed Mushrooms

(Calories: 124; Fat: 2g; Carbs: 17g; Protein: 12g)

Dinner

Turkey Potato Casserole W/Eggplant and Tomato

(Calories: 278; Fat: 2.6g; Carbs: 15g; Protein: 28g)

Dessert

Mango Chia Seed Pudding

(Calories: 146; Fat: 26g; Carbs: 15g; Protein: 23g)

Day 7(Totals: Calories: 886; Fat: 72g; Carbs: 78g; Protein: 36.9g)

Breakfast:

Coconut Flour Pancakes

(Calories: 65; Fat: 4.2g; Carbs: 3.6g; Protein: 2.5g)

Snack

Eggplant Caponata

(Calories: 98; Fat: 2.18g; Carbs: 19g; Protein: 3g)

Lunch

Lettuce Tacos With Chipotle Chicken

(Calories: 175; Fat: 0g; Carbs: 3; Protein: 10g)

Snack

Sautéed Mushrooms

(Calories: 124; Fat: 2g; Carbs: 17g; Protein: 12g)

Dinner

Turkey Potato Casserole W/Eggplant and Tomato

(Calories: 278; Fat: 2.6g; Carbs: 15g; Protein: 28g)

Dessert

Mango Chia Seed Pudding

(Calories: 146; Fat: 26g; Carbs: 15g; Protein: 23g)

Week 2: Shopping List and Meal Plan

- Chicken Sausage, Pepperoni, Marinara, Tomatoes, Onion
- Mushroom, Black Olives, Oregano, Garlic Powder, Salt
- Yellow Onion, Turkey , Roasted Onion, Pumpkin Puree
- Chicken Broth, Honey, Chili Spice, Sea Salt, Cinnamon
- Coconut Milk, Eggs, Blueberries, Shredded Coconut
- Potato, Olive Oil, Mushrooms, Italian Sausage
- Beef, Coconut Oil, Green Olive, Drained Capers
- Brine, Iceberg Lettuce, Bacon, Avocado, Tomato
- Mayonnaise, Cocoa, Honey, Pure vanilla extract, Pumpkin Puree
- Almond Butter, Maple Syrup, Nutmeg, Ginger, Butter
- Olive Oil, White Wine, Radishes, Balsamic Vinegar

Day 1 (Totals: Calories: 1034; Fat: 58g; Carbs: 68g; Protein: 38g)

Breakfast:

Sweet Potato Muffins

(Calories: 100; Fat: 5g; Carbs: 10g; Protein: 6g)

Snack

Eggplant Caponata

(Calories: 175; Fat: 0g; Carbs: 3g; Protein: 10g)

Lunch

Spicy Picadillo Lettuce Wrap

(Calories: 178; Fat: 7.8g; Carbs: 7.8g; Protein: 20.5g)

Snack

Sautéed Mushrooms

(Calories: 124; Fat: 2g; Carbs: 17g; Protein: 12g)

Dinner

Pizza Soup

(Calories: 323; Fat: 19g; Carbs: 15g; Protein: 12g)

Dessert

Chocolaty Cocoa Mousse

(Calories: 134; Fat: 3.8g; Carbs: 6; Protein: 8g)

Day 2 (Totals: Calories: 725; Fat: 82g; Carbs: 57g; Protein, 54g)

Breakfast:

Blueberry Coconut French Toast

(Calories: 111; Fat: 8g; Carbohydrate: 5g; Protein: 5.5g)

Snack

Perfectly Sautéed Mushroom

(Calories: 124; Fat: 2g; Carbohydrate: 17g; Protein: 12g)

Lunch

California Turkey, Bacon Lettuce Wrap With Basil Mayo

(Calories: 150; Fat: 13.35g; Carbs: 17.5; Protein: 4g)

Snack

Sautéed Mushrooms

(Calories: 124; Fat: 2g; Carbs: 17g; Protein: 12g)

Dinner

Roasted Heirloom Carrots

(Calories: 70; Fat: 3g; Carbs: 11g; Protein: 1g)

Dessert

Mango Chia Seed Pudding

(Calories: 146; Fat: 26g; Carbs: 15g; Protein: 23g)

Day 3 (Totals: Calories: 1034; Fat: 58g; Carbs, 68g; Protein: 38g)

Breakfast:

Sweet Potato Muffins

(Calories: 100; Fat: 5g; Carbs: 10g; Protein: 6g)

Snack

Eggplant Caponata

(Calories: 175; Fat: 0g; Carbs: 3g; Protein: 10g)

Lunch

Spicy Picadillo Lettuce Wrap

(Calories: 178; Fat: 7.8g; Carbs: 7.8g; Protein: 20.5g)

Snack

Sautéed Mushrooms

(Calories: 124; Fat: 2g; Carbs: 17g; Protein: 12g)

Dinner

Pizza Soup

(Calories: 323; Fat: 19g; Carbs: 15g; Protein: 12g)

Dessert

Chocolaty Cocoa Mousse

(Calories: 134; Fat: 3.8g; Carbs: 6; Protein: 8g)

Day 4 (Totals: Calories: 725; Fat: 82g; Carbs: 57g; Protein: 54g)

Breakfast:

Blueberry Coconut French Toast

(Calories: 111; Fat: 8g; Carbs: 5g; Protein: 5.5g)

Snack

Sautéed Mushrooms

(Calories: 124; Fat: 2g; Carbs: 17g; Protein: 12g)

Lunch

California Turkey, Bacon Lettuce Wrap With Basil Mayo

(Calories: 150; Fat: 13.35g; Carbs: 17.5; Protein: 4g)

Snack

Sautéed Mushrooms

(Calories: 124; Fat: 2g; Carbs: 17g; Protein: 12g)

Dinner

Roasted Heirloom Carrots

(Calories: 70; Fat: 3g; Carbs: 11g; Protein: 1g)

Dessert

Mango Chia Seed Pudding

(Calories: 146; Fat: 26g; Carbs: 15g; Protein: 23g)

Day 5 (Totals: Calories: 1034; Fat: 58g; Carbs: 68g; Protein: 38G)

Breakfast:

Sweet Potato Muffins

(Calories: 100; Fat: 5g; Carbs: 10g; Protein: 6g)

Snack

Eggplant Caponata

(Calories: 175; Fat: 0g; Carbs: 3g; Protein: 10g)

Lunch

Spicy Picadillo Lettuce Wrap

(Calories: 178; Fat: 7.8g; Carbs: 7.8g; Protein: 20.5g)

Snack

Sautéed Mushrooms

(Calories: 124; Fat: 2g; Carbs: 17g; Protein: 12g)

Dinner

Pizza Soup

(Calories: 323; Fat: 19g; Carbs: 15g; Protein: 12g)

Dessert

Chocolaty Cocoa Mousse

(Calories: 134; Fat: 3.8g; Carbohydrate: 6; Protein: 8g)

Day 6 (Totals: Calories: 725; Fat: 82g; Carbs: 57g protein; Protein: 54g)

Breakfast:

Blueberry Coconut French Toast

(Calories: 111; Fat: 8g; Carbs: 5g; Protein: 5.5g)

Snack

Sautéed Mushrooms

(Calories: 124; Fat: 2g; Carbs: 17g; Protein: 12g)

Lunch

California Turkey, Bacon Lettuce Wrap With Basil Mayo

(Calories: 150; Fat: 13.35g; Carbs: 17.5; Protein: 4g)

Snack

Sautéed Mushrooms

(Calories: 124; Fat: 2g; Carbs: 17g; Protein: 12g)

Dinner

Roasted Heirloom Carrots

(Calories: 70; Fat: 3g; Carbs: 11g; Protein: 1g)

Dessert

Mango Chia Seed Pudding

(Calories: 146; Fat: 26g; Carbs: 15g; Protein: 23g)

Day 7 (Totals: Calories: 725; Fat: 82g; Carbs: 57g; Protein: 54g)

Breakfast:

Blueberry Coconut French Toast

(Calories: 111; Fat: 8g; Carbs: 5g; Protein: 5.5g)

Snack

Sautéed Mushrooms

(Calories: 124; Fat: 2g; Carbs: 17g; Protein: 12g)

Lunch

California Turkey, Bacon Lettuce Wrap With Basil Mayo

(Calories: 150; Fat: 13.35g; Carbs: 17.5; Protein: 4g)

Snack

Sautéed Mushrooms

(Calories: 124; Fat: 2g; Carbs: 17g; Protein: 12g)

Dinner

Roasted Heirloom Carrots

(Calories: 70; Fat: 3g; Carbs: 11g; Protein: 1g)

Dessert

Mango Chia Seed Pudding

(Calories: 146; Fat: 26g; Carbs: 15g; Protein: 23g)

Week 3: Shopping List and Meal Plan

- Bananas, Almond Butter, Coconut Flour, Cinnamon
- Baking Powder, Pure vanilla extract, Salt, Dark Chocolate
- Extra Virgin Coconut Oil, Raw Honey, Large Eggs, Coconut Milk
- Pure vanilla extract, Coconut Milk, Tartar Cream, Baking Soda
- Sea Salt, Carrots, Bell Peppers, Onion, Garlic, Cumin Seeds
- Avocado, Lime, Salsa, Roma Tomatoes, Cucumber, Cilantro

- Spinach, Nitrate Free Bacon, Butternut Squash, Sage, Paprika
- Pepper, Turkey, Sweet Potatoes, Eggplant, Chili Powder
- Oregano, Cardamom, Tarragon Flakes, Almond Milk, Rosemary

Day 1 (Totals: Calories: 1238; Fat: 63g; Carbs: 37.8g; Protein: 48g)

Breakfast:

Chocolate Chunk Banana Bread

(Calories: 250; Fat: 18.2g; Carbs: 19.4g; Protein: 6.8g)

Snack

Balsamic Rosemary Roasted Vegetables

(Calories: 98; Fat: 2.18g; Carbs: 19g; Protein: 3g)

Lunch

Taco Salad In Mason Jar

(Calories: 177; Fat: 9.14g; Carbs: 9.8g; Protein: 16g)

Snack

Crispy Carrot Chips

(Calories: 280; Fat: 0g; Carbs: 0g; Protein: 0g)

Dinner

Skillet Chicken Thighs With Butternut Squash

(Calories: 323; Fat: 19g; Carbs: 15g; Protein: 12g)

Dessert

Graham Crackers

(Calories: 110; Fat: 0g; Carbs: 10; Protein: 0g)

Day 2 (Totals: Calories: 886; Fat: 72g; Carbs: 78g; protein: 36.9)

Breakfast:

Coconut Flour Pancakes

(Calories: 65; Fat: 4.2g; Carbs: 3.6g; Protein: 2.5g)

Snack

Eggplant Caponata

(Calories: 98; Fat: 2.18g; Carbs: 19g; Protein: 3g)

Lunch

Lettuce Tacos With Chipotle Chicken

(Calories: 175; Fat: 0g; Carbs: 3; Protein: 10g)

Snack

Sautéed Mushrooms

(Calories: 124; Fat: 2g; Carbs: 17g; Protein: 12g)

Dinner

Sweet Potato Turkey Casserole W/Eggplant and Tomato

(Calories: 278; Fat: 2.6g; Carbs: 15g; Protein: 28g)

Dessert

Mango Chia Seed Pudding

(Calories: 146; Fat: 26g; Carbs: 15g; Protein: 23g)

Day 3 (Totals: Calories: 1238; Fat: 63g; Carbs: 37.8g; Protein: 48g)

Breakfast:

Chocolate Chunk Banana Bread

(Calories: 250; Fat: 18.2g; Carbs: 19.4g; Protein: 6.8g)

Snack

Balsamic Rosemary Roasted Vegetables

(Calories: 98; Fat: 2.18g; Carbs: 19g; Protein: 3g)

Lunch

Taco Salad In Mason Jar

(Calories: 177; Fat: 9.14g; Carbs: 9.8g; Protein: 16g)

Snack

Crispy Carrot Chips

(Calories: 280; Fat: 0g; Carbs: 0g; Protein: 0g)

Dinner

Skillet Chicken Thighs With Butternut Squash

(Calories: 323; Fat: 19g; Carbs: 15g; Protein: 12g)

Dessert

Graham Crackers

(Calories: 110; Fat: 0g; Carbs: 10; Protein: 0g)

Day 4 (Totals: Calories: 886; Fat: 72g; Carbs: 78g; Protein: 36.9)

Breakfast:

Coconut Flour Pancakes

(Calories: 65; Fat: 4.2g; Carbs: 3.6g; Protein: 2.5g)

Snack

Eggplant Caponata

(Calories: 98; Fat: 2.18g; Carbs: 19g; Protein: 3g)

Lunch

Lettuce Tacos With Chipotle Chicken

(Calories: 175; Fat: 0g; Carbs: 3; Protein: 10g)

Snack

Sautéed Mushrooms

(Calories: 124; Fat: 2g; Carbs: 17g; Protein: 12g)

Dinner

Sweet Potato Turkey Casserole W/Eggplant and Tomato

(Calories: 278; Fat: 2.6g; Carbs: 15g; Protein: 28g)

Dessert

Mango Chia Seed Pudding

(Calories: 146; Fat: 26g; Carbs: 15g; Protein: 23g)

Day 5 (Totals: Calories: 1238; Fat: 63g; Carbs: 37.8g; Protein: 48g)

Breakfast:

Chocolate Chunk Banana Bread

(Calories: 250; Fat: 18.2g; Carbs: 19.4g; Protein: 6.8g)

Snack

Balsamic Rosemary Roasted Vegetables

(Calories: 98; Fat: 2.18g; Carbs: 19g; Protein: 3g)

Lunch

Taco Salad In Mason Jar

(Calorie: 177; Fat: 9.14g; Carbs: 9.8g; Protein: 16g)

Snack

Crispy Carrot Chips

(Calories: 280; Fat: 0g; Carbs: 0g; Protein: 0g)

Dinner

Skillet Chicken Thighs With Butternut Squash

(Calories: 323; Fat: 19g; Carbs: 15g; Protein: 12g)

Dessert

Graham Crackers

(Calories: 110; Fat: 0g; Carbs: 10; Protein: 0g)

Day 6 (Totals: Calories: 886; Fat: 72g; Carbs: 78g; Protein, 36.9g)

Breakfast:

Coconut Flour Pancakes

(Calories: 65; Fat: 4.2g; Carbs: 3.6g; Protein: 2.5g)

Snack

Eggplant Caponata

(Calories: 98; Fat: 2.18g; Carbs: 19g; Protein: 3g)

Lunch

Lettuce Tacos With Chipotle Chicken

(Calories: 175; Fat: 0g; Carbs: 3g; Protein: 10g)

Snack

Sautéed Mushrooms

(Calories: 124; Fat: 2g; Carbs: 17g; Protein: 12g)

Dinner

Sweet Potato Turkey Casserole W/Eggplant and Tomato

(Calories: 278; Fat: 2.6g; Carbs: 15g; Protein: 28g)

Dessert

Mango Chia Seed Pudding

(Calorie: 146; Fat: 26g; Carbs: 15g; Protein: 23g)

Day 7 (Totals: Calories: 886; Fat: 72g; Carbs: 78g; Protein, 38.9g)

Breakfast:

Coconut Flour Pancakes

(Calories: 65; Fat: 4.2g; Carbs: 3.6g; Protein: 2.5g)

Snack

Eggplant Caponata

(Calories: 98; Fat: 2.18g; Carbs: 19g; Protein: 3g)

Lunch

Lettuce Tacos With Chipotle Chicken

(Calorie: 175; Fat: 0g; Carbs: 3g; Protein: 10g)

Snack

Sautéed Mushrooms

(Calories: 124; Fat: 2g; Carbs: 17g; Protein: 12g)

Dinner

Sweet Potato Turkey Casserole W/Eggplant and Tomato

(Calories: 278; Fat: 2.6g; Carbs: 15g; Protein: 28g)

Dessert

Mango Chia Seed Pudding

(Calories: 146; Fat: 26g; Carbs: 15g; Protein: 23g)

Week 4: Shopping List and Meal Plan

- Chicken Sausage, Pepperoni, Marinara, Tomatoes, Onion
- Mushroom, Black Olives, Oregano, Garlic Powder, Salt

- Yellow Onion, Turkey, Roasted Onion, Pumpkin Puree
- Chicken Broth, Honey, Chili Spice, Sea Salt, Cinnamon
- Coconut Milk, Eggs, Blueberries, Shredded Coconut
- Potatoes, Olive Oil, Mushrooms, Italian Sausage, Beef, Coconut Oil
- Green Olives, Drained Capers, Brine, Iceberg Lettuce, Bacon
- Avocado, Tomato, Mayonnaise, Cocoa, Honey, Pure vanilla extract
- Pumpkin Puree, Almond Butter, Maple Syrup, Nutmeg
- Ginger, Butter, Olive Oil, White Wine, Radishes, White Balsamic

Day 1 (Totals: Calories: 1034; Fat: 58g; Carbs: 68g; Protein: 38g)

Breakfast:

Sweet Potato Muffins

(Calories: 100; Fat: 5g; Carbs: 10g; Protein: 6g)

Snack

Eggplant Caponata

(Calories: 175; Fat: 0g; Carbs: 3g; Protein: 10g)

Lunch

Spicy Picadillo Lettuce Wrap

(Calories: 178; Fat: 7.8g; Carbs: 7.8g; Protein: 20.5g)

Snack

Sautéed Mushrooms

(Calories: 124; Fat: 2g; Carbs: 17g; Protein: 12g)

Dinner

Pizza Soup

(Calories: 323; Fat: 19g; Carbs: 15g; Protein: 12g)

Dessert

Chocolaty Cocoa Mousse

(Calories: 134; Fat: 3.8g; Carbs: 6; Protein: 8g)

Day 2 (Totals: Calories: 725; Fat: 82g; Carbs: 57g; Protein: 54g)

Breakfast:

Blueberry Coconut French Toast

(Calories: 111; Fat: 8g; Carbs: 5g; Protein: 5.5g)

Snack

Sautéed Mushrooms

(Calories: 124; Fat: 2g; Carbs: 17g; Protein: 12g)

Lunch

California Turkey, Bacon Lettuce Wrap With Basil Mayo

(Calories: 150; Fat: 13.35g; Carbs: 17.5; Protein: 4g)

Snack

Eggplant Caponata

(Calories: 175; Fat: 0g; Carbs: 3g; Protein: 10g)

Dinner

Roasted Heirloom Carrots

(Calories: 70; Fat: 3g; Carbs: 11g; Protein: 1g)

Dessert

Mango Chia Seed Pudding

(Calories: 146; Fat: 26g; Carbs: 15g; Protein: 23g)

Day 3(Totals: Calories: 1034; Fat: 58g; Carbs: 68g; Protein: 38g)

Breakfast:

Sweet Potato Muffins

(Calories: 100; Fat: 5g; Carbs: 10g; Protein: 6g)

Snack

Eggplant Caponata

(Calories: 175; Fat: 0g; Carbs: 3g; Protein: 10g)

Lunch

Spicy Picadillo Lettuce Wrap

(Calories: 178; Fat: 7.8g; Carbs: 7.8g; Protein: 20.5g)

Snack

Sautéed Mushrooms

(Calories: 124; Fat: 2g; Carbs: 17g; Protein: 12g)

Dinner

Pizza Soup

(Calories: 323; Fat: 19g; Carbs: 15g; Protein: 12g)

Dessert

Chocolaty Cocoa Mousse

(Calories: 134; Fat: 3.8g; Carbs: 6g; Protein: 3.8g)

Day 4(Totals: Calories: 725; Fat: 82g; Carbs: 57g; Protein: 54g)

Breakfast:

Blueberry Coconut French Toast

(Calories: 111; Fat: 8g; Carbs: 5g; Protein: 5.5g)

Snack

Sautéed Mushrooms

(Calories: 124; Fat: 2g; Carbs: 17g; Protein: 12g)

Lunch

California Turkey, Bacon Lettuce Wrap With Basil Mayo

(Calories: 150; Fat: 13.35g; Carbs: 17.5; Protein: 4g)

Snack

Eggplant Caponata

(Calories: 175; Fat: 0g; Carbs: 3g; Protein: 10g)

Dinner

Roasted Heirloom Carrots

(Calories: 70; Fat: 3g; Carbs: 11g; Protein: 1g)

Dessert

Mango Chia Seed Pudding

(Calories: 146; Fat: 26g; Carbs: 15g; Protein: 23g)

Day 5 (Totals: Calories: 1034; Fat: 58g; Carbs: 68g; Protein: 38g)

Breakfast:

Sweet Potato Muffins

(Calories: 100; Fat: 5g; Carbs: 10g; Protein: 6g)

Snack

Eggplant Caponata

(Calories: 175; Fat: 0g; Carbs: 3g; Protein: 10g)

Lunch

Spicy Picadillo Lettuce Wrap

(Calories: 178; Fat: 7.8g; Carbs: 7.8g; Protein: 20.5g)

Snack

Sautéed Mushrooms

(Calories: 124; Fat: 2g; Carbs: 17g; Protein: 12g)

Dinner

Pizza Soup

(Calories: 323; Fat: 19g; Carbs: 15g; Protein: 12g)

Dessert

Chocolaty Cocoa Mousse

(Calories: 134; Fat: 3.8g; Carbs: 6; Protein: 3.8g)

Day 6(Totals: Calories: 725; Fat: 82g; Carbs: 57g; Protein: 54g)

Breakfast:

Blueberry Coconut French Toast

(Calories: 111; Fat: 8g; Carbs: 5g; Protein: 5.5g)

Snack

Sautéed Mushrooms

(Calories: 124; Fat: 2g; Carbs: 17g; Protein: 12g)

Lunch

California Turkey, Bacon Lettuce Wrap With Basil Mayo

(Calories: 150; Fat: 13.35g; Carbs: 17.5; Protein: 4g)

Snack

Eggplant Caponata

(Calories: 175; Fat: 0g; Carbs: 3g; Protein: 10g)

Dinner

Roasted Heirloom Carrots

(Calories: 70; Fat: 3g; Carbs: 11g; Protein: 1g)

Dessert

Mango Chia Seed Pudding

(Calories: 146; Fat: 26g; Carbs: 15g; Protein: 23g)

Day 7(Totals: Calories: 724; Fat: 82g; Carbs: 57g; Protein: 54g)

Breakfast:

Blueberry Coconut French Toast

(Calories: 111; Fat: 8g; Carbs: 5g; Protein: 5.5g)

Snack

Sautéed Mushrooms

(Calories: 124; Fat: 2g; Carbs: 17g; Protein: 12g)

Lunch

California Turkey, Bacon Lettuce Wrap With Basil Mayo

(Calories: 150; Fat: 13.35g; Carbs: 17.5; Protein: 4g)

Snack

Eggplant Caponata

(Calories: 175; Fat: 0g; Carbs: 3g; Protein: 10g)

Dinner

Heirloom Carrots

(Calories: 70; Fat: 3g; Carbs: 11g; Protein: 1g)

Dessert

Mango Chia Seed Pudding

(Calories: 146; Fat: 26g; Carbs: 15g; Protein: 23g)

Conclusion

Once again, I would like to thank you for having the patience of reading it fully.

I do hope you had just as much fun reading and experimenting with the recipes as much as I enjoyed writing the book.

Stay safe, Stay healthy and God Bless!

Printed in Great Britain
by Amazon